Defeating Breast Cancer

ON-LINE VIDEO
COURSE AVAILABLE

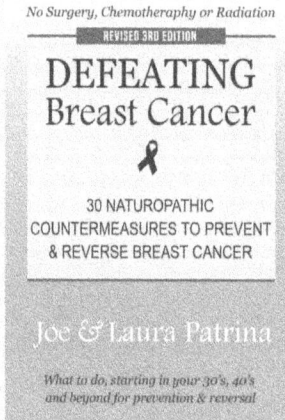

No Surgery, Chemotheraphy or Radiation

REVISED 3RD EDITION

DEFEATING
Breast Cancer

30 NATUROPATHIC
COUNTERMEASURES TO PREVENT
& REVERSE BREAST CANCER

Joe & Laura Patrina

What to do, starting in your 30's, 40's and beyond for prevention & reversal

Welcome to *Defeating Breast Cancer*, a narrative-based journal presenting the year Laura dramatically shrunk her cancer tumors, *solely* through naturopathic means.

We recommend that you read the book narrative first, as like the authors, the reader may also be on a quest for courage and alternatives, just as we were. To dig deeper, a 35-segment On-line Video Course program is available as a Web-delivered educational series.

The online program, presents key findings subject- by-subject, providing the viewer a direct-action plan for their situation, whether preventative or as a component of treatment. The video program can be previewed on the *DefeatingCancerNaturally.com* website.

As a thank-you for buying the book, go to *DefeatingCancerNaturally.com/Book* for a free PDF titled: BLUNTING VIRAL ATTACKS – describing what to do with both cancer and Covid-19 viral threats. As you will find, the overlap between cancer and viruses is a key factor to prevention and reversal.

Joe & Laura Patrina

Acknowledgements

Doctor David Bronstein and Doctor Russel Blaylock are two MDs who taught us many of the key findings in this book. They each publish a monthly newsletter, which one can order online from *NewsmaxHealth.com*, and I have read all of their work for many years now. Naturopath MD practitioners, completely grounded in traditional medicine know-how, they compliment this with tireless research on the latest "root cause" breakthroughs and natural treatments. They will be quoted here and there throughout the journal. I am particularly grateful for their insights on the role of iodine in preventing breast cancer (Dr. Bronstein has a book on this) and the viral causes of cancer (which Dr. Blaylock covers in detail in his Vol. 16, No. 2 publication).

Doctor Robert Bard has been watching over Laura for five years with his non-invasive sonograms and other advanced imaging systems, tracking Laura's breast and lymph node health. Dr. Bard also clued us into the issues of dense breast tissue and the role of inflammation in driving cancer.

Doctor Mark Breiner educated us on toxicity and rid Laura of carcinogen deposits that had accumulated over the course of a lifetime.

Doctor Joseph Raffaele cared for Laura's internal hormonal chemistry, educated us on many aspects of cellular biology, and described breakthrough findings about cancer cell wall receptors – which in turn led to a natural treatment that isolates cancer cells from hormonal contact and stimulus.

Doctors Cheryl Vincent and Stephen Karpenko, our Naturopaths and Nutritionists who guided us with ideas, supplements and dosages.

Joe Patrina
Researcher, 2019

ISBN: 978-1-7330672-6-3   [Paperback Edition]

Please visit *hoodwinked.net* for video versions of this manuscript.
Printed and bound in The United States of America.

Published by LittleHouse Enterprises Inc.

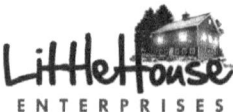

READ THIS FIRST

Disclaimer

*This account of how Laura's cancer tumors disappeared is not a promise or endorsement that guarantees or warrants the same results for others. **Defeating Breast Cancer** describes what Laura did, and it explains the reasoning behind why she did these things. No claim is cited as proven. Assertions are solely our internal and personal view on the possible explanations of why our actions may have worked. We share these personal insights with you merely as background and not as a prescription. Neither Laura nor Joe are medical doctors; nor have we taken any formal course of study in preparing this book. In any action taken regarding your health, you are urged to use your own best counsel and judgment, including discussions with cancer medical doctor specialists and nutritionists.*

Personal Statement

*"In 2014 I was diagnosed with breast cancer. At that moment, I faced a world where women are never told how to prevent breast cancer, nor given many options in how to treat it; they are instead rushed into operating rooms. Once diagnosed, my self-healing plan evolved by tapping into the know-how of many traditional and naturopath doctors. My husband and I combined the **extensive knowledge of experts**, connected the dots, and thus avoided invasive surgery, radiation, and chemotherapy. With self-healing, my tumors shrank by half in three months with no sign of tumors at year's end and no regrowth at the end of year five."*

~ **Laura**

You Will Learn How to Disrupt Breast Cancer ...

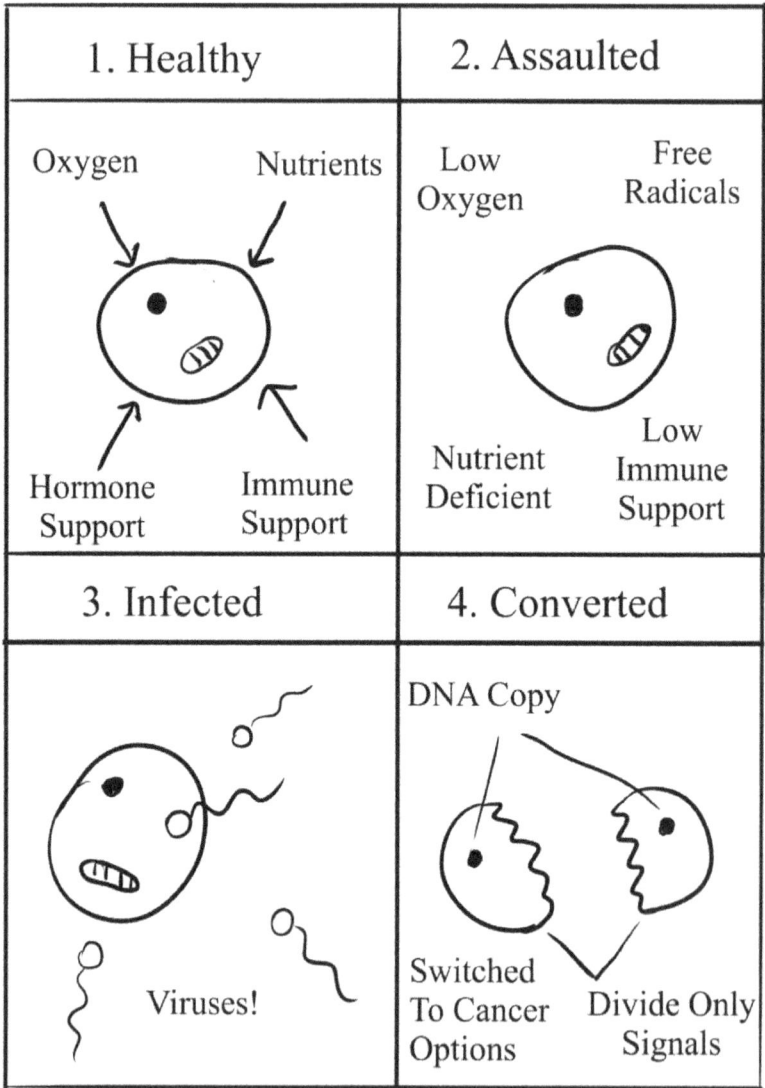

... Along Each Stage
of Its Expansion Path

5. Tumor Formed	6. Agression
2, 4, 8, 16... Billions 8 Years	Inflammation Drivers Divide Divide Divide
7. Dominance	8. Spreading
Blood Vessel Provisions Sugar Sugar Sugar	New Tumors Metastisis

Contents

Laura's Note

I want to share something with you... it's how to overcome the dread of breast cancer, the dread of surgery, radiation, and chemotherapy.

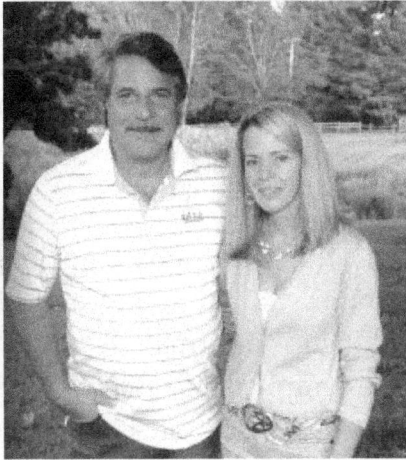

Authors Joe & Laura Patrina

In 2014, I was diagnosed with breast cancer tumors. Once my husband Joe and I decided to tackle the tumors using organic, self-healing methods, our children urged Joe to keep a journal of everything we researched, every medical meeting we attended, and every element of the organic approach we assembled. We believe self-healing is straightforward:

Diet:	Deprive cancer, as it needs 16x as much sugar as do normal cells. Instead feed the body ketones.
Tumor Infiltration:	Degrade tumors via supplements to disrupt cell division. Slow them down, sicken them!
Immune System Empowerment:	Eliminate toxins and feed immune cells the vitamins they require to attack weakened tumors 24/7. Kill visible and invisible cancer colonies throughout the body.

A year later, with the tumors no longer appearing on the mammogram, women young and old soon began contacting us looking for information and to possibly share in our solution. Joe compiled his research journal into a draft manuscript, and we sent PDF files out to women recently diagnosed. Joe continued taking notes for four more years while we kept watch on my status with Doctor Robert Bard at the Bard Cancer Center, an advanced, noninvasive, cancer diagnostics facility in New York City.

Finally, after five years, we decided the time had come to release the book, and we titled it *Defeating Breast Cancer – 30 Naturopathic Countermeasures to Prevent and Reverse Breast*

Cancer. Then in 2019, to complement the book, we produced the *Preventing & Defeating Breast Cancer – On-line Program*, 32 videos teaching women how to lower the dread of breast cancer by using the expertise we had gleaned to manage health.

Within the self-healing plan, women can follow many different courses of action to prevent and reverse occurrences of breast cancer, and we list suggestions of what to do to prevent it in your thirties, what to consider in your forties as women become more vulnerable, and what to do if diagnosed or even in recovery.

Defeating Breast Cancer speaks unfiltered. The ideas and decisions prevailing over the course of five years — even the "far out" ones — are reflected just as experienced.

Laura and Joe Patrina,
parents of four, live in Connecticut.

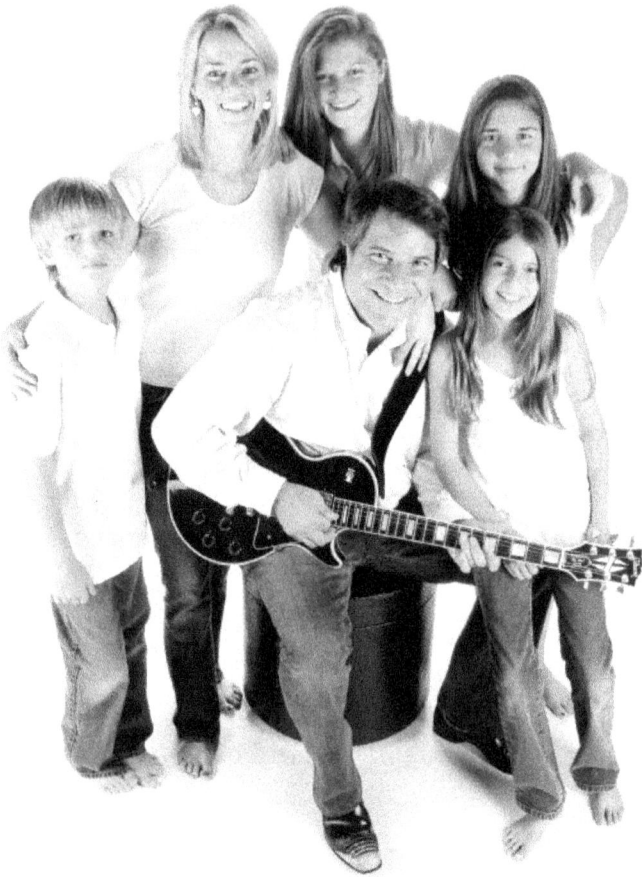

- *Women Now Have a Choice*

- *What You Will Learn*

Women Now Have a Choice

*T*he truth stands that one-in-eight women develop breast cancer and that black women have an even higher chance of tumor formation. But can't we offer better counsel than the standard "don't smoke, don't drink, and get regular exercise" advice one hears over and over again?

I, a mother of four and a black-belt karate instructor, survived breast cancer... and I did it naturopathically. Formulated through research and the insight of many traditional and naturopath practitioners, the thirty elements of the self-healing program shrank my tumors in months with no sign of tumors at year's end and no regrowth at the end of year five.

Whatever your current situation is, my advice stands: Don't wait to educate yourself. Women need to dig into the ways of breast cancer long before it has a chance to catch them by surprise. Instead, you surprise it! *Defeating Breast Cancer* teaches how to stay ahead of the curve. Fear gets demoted, putting women in the driver's seat. But you must act early.

The thirty self-healing action steps fall within the three principle rails mentioned earlier:

Diet:	Deprive cancer, as it needs 16x as much sugar as do normal cells. Instead feed the body ketones.
Tumor Infiltration:	Degrade tumors via supplements to disrupt cell division. Slow them down, sicken them!
Immune System Empowerment:	Eliminate toxins and feed immune cells the vitamins they require to attack weakened tumors 24/7. Kill visible and invisible cancer colonies throughout the body.

From here, many interesting insights and practical advice follow, which are all presented in the *Defeating Breast Cancer* book. As background, in 2014, medical professionals diagnosed me with two breast cancer tumors. Just before my diagnosis as you might recall, Angelina Jolie, the American icon, decided to have both of her breasts removed *as a precaution!* Women walk the gangplank simply hearing the words "breast cancer" with brutal surgery becoming the response *du jour*—and I assumed the same for myself.

Well, I, the mother hen, while sitting in the surgeon's office dared to ask, "How long have these tumors been growing?" He (most breast surgeons are male) admitted that the tumors had been growing for eight to ten years. Right then I put the brakes on refusing to sign up for the surgery that he was urging me to schedule for the very next week. If it had taken years for the tumors to get to where things now stood, I could wait a bit longer before losing a breast! Instead, I decided to try self-healing *and to try it for just three months.* When family members learned of my decision, they immediately protested saying things such as, "Stop screwing around and get the things cut out!"

After three months, my tumors shrank by 50 percent. It took one year to declare a guarded victory, and a second, third, fourth, and fifth year to be sure as I had periodic sonogram and mammogram tests along the way. Afterward, my husband Joe and I arranged the thirty steps of the plan into a prevention sequence one could adopt—starting as early as in your late twenties —to thwart the development of cancer as you age.

Most cancers take eight to fifteen years to incubate before becoming visible. The easiest of the thirty elements, "nipping outbreaks in the bud," certainly can be put to work early. We also developed the *Defeating Breast Cancer* video series to accompany the book, which is intended to help coach the reader in digesting all of the findings.

Briefly, let's look at the 30 prevention steps, described in detail throughout the book.

In Your Twenties and Thirties — You Want to Prevent Cancer Formation — and need to keep your immune system empowered and able to eliminate periodic mutations. Here are the highlights:

1. Maintain a low-sugar, low-carb diet

2. Correct thyroid/iodine deficiency

3. Eliminate toxins accumulated since birth

4. Treat dense breast tissue by using primrose and serraflazyme enzyme that dissolve scar tissue.

5. Take vitamins C, D and E daily.

6. Get regular exercise, don't smoke, drink alcohol in moderation

In Your Forties—It's Time to Stymie Unseen Cancer Colonies. A breast cancer can take years to grow large enough to be detected. Add further measures that thwart budding *unseen* colonies, slow down cell division rates and allow the immune system time to counter them. These measures include:

7. Periodic cleanses

8. Take green tea concentrate supplements to plug cancer receptors

9. Testing for and eliminating allergies

10. Nutritional testing and supplementation

11. Taking omega-3 and resveratrol for the heart

12. Take Curcumin and Boswellia extracts as anti-viral, anti-inflammatory measures

13. Drinking green tea concentrate to plug cancer receptors

14. Taking evening hot sea salt baths to activate the immune system

15. Taking beta-glucan and red Reishe mushroom extracts for immune support

16. Enhancing your supplementation of antioxygens

17. Using copaiba oil to calm chronic inflammation

18. Taking probiotics to strengthen digestion

19. Exercising regularly, no smoking, and drinking alcohol in moderation

If Diagnosed—You Can Overwhelm Visible Cancer Occurrences. Once your cancer is visible, you can add another layer of dietary, supplementary, and environmental measures to overwhelm the tumor(s). Some highlights of these measures include:

20. Infiltrate the Tumor with alkaline baking soda infused in honey

21. Eating zero-sugar, zero-carbs, and zero-animal fats for three-plus months

22. Testing for and treating diabetes to reduce standing glucose levels

23. Using CBD oil infused with frankincense to slow cancer division rates

24. Drinking double-helix water to boost the body's overall energy charge

25. Using infrared light to "unclump" blood cells, promoting oxygen

26. Adopting and strictly following a low-stress lifestyle to temper cortisol/sugar spikes

27. Taking B vitamins for the nervous system to stem anxiety and to calm you

28. Making sleep a priority, allowing the immune system time to work

29. Take Curcumin to inhibit vascular support for budding tumors

30. Regular exercise, no smoking, and absolutely NO drinking of alcohol, as alcohol supplies tumors with estrogen

Should you be diagnosed with cancer, periodic and harmless sonogram images will determine any rate of progress so that you can stick to the organic plan without dread of the unknown, and you can always enlist medical intervention if necessary. And because breast cancer has a way of returning, survivors may want to explore self-healing to improve their chances. As the title of this section, "Women Now Have a Choice," states women can choose to empower themselves to make self-care their first option with medical intervention sitting on the back burner until needed. Let choice overcome chance.

But there is much to learn.

What You Will Learn

*T*o understand why the thirty self-healing steps work, you must dig into the nuts and bolts of the *Defeating Breast Cancer* book and the *Defeating Breast Cancer* videos. But to give you a feel for the tactics of this naturopath approach, this section "What You Will Learn," summarizes some of the plan's key elements. Let's get started by touching upon the three key topics of the book: *diet, tumor infiltration, and immune system empowerment.*

Diet—You Will Learn about Starving Cancer because Cancer *Craves* Sugar

You will find the expanded explanation of why cancer craves sugar in the body of this book. Here, we will simply say that healthy cells create energy by combining oxygen and sugar, called *oxidation*, similar to burning logs on a fire, whereas cancer cells hide from oxygen and instead create their energy by *fermenting* large quantities of sugar as does a whisky still.

Cancer cells require sixteen times as much sugar than normal cells to achieve this.

The diet centerpiece for defeating cancer seeks to provide the body with just enough sugar for healthy cells while leaving cancer tumors high and dry. The day you start with such a diet is the day the cancer cells begin to go hungry. As the weeks go by, and the body's hidden sugar reserves dwindle, tumor cells slowly die of starvation. The rest of the body, however, does fine without all that sugar. Using fats, your liver creates a substitute energy packet called "ketones", and healthy cells can digest ketones, but cancer cannot. This fuel switch, therefore – from sugars to ketones – isolates the cancer.

Diet – You Will Learn How to Identify Food Allergies and Missing Nutrients

Most diets contain foods that you are allergic to so you must avoid them. Most diets are also missing foods that supply essential nutrients. You need to sort out these mismatches or else hobble along like a car using the wrong gas.

Diet – You Will Learn that Cancer Hates Alkalinity

Alkalinity allows for optimum levels of oxygen to be transported to the cells, a healthy condition. Conversely, cancer cells shun oxygen and instead prefer an acidic, low-oxygen environment. Although the blood pH does not change, the pH in the cells and intracellular space becomes more acidic. So, in order to deprive cancer cells, in addition to controlling sugars, you must gravitate toward foods that result in greater cellular alkalinity. The matrix of sugar and acidic foods versus non-sugar and alkaline foods is presented in the main body of the book.

Diet — You Will Learn about the Diabetes and Cancer Connection

As explained later in the book, *diabetes* — excess sugar in the blood — is an aid to cancer tumors as extended periods of blood sugar give cancer ample time to extract all the sugar it needs from the bloodstream. Therefore, besides dealing with cancer, you must simultaneously deal with diabetes, too. Both conditions involve bodily processes weakened by age, but you can offset these weaknesses via supplementation.

Infiltration and Empowerment — You Will Learn how to Poison Cancer and Boost Your Immune System

Eventually, the tumor fizzles out. But the time needed for this milestone depends upon the size of the tumor; complemented by the use of *tumor infiltration* or "poisoning" tactics that further weaken the nutrient-deprived tumor; and *immune system empowerment* via detoxing and using specific nutrients to help immune cells kill off weakened tumors in an accelerated manner.

Let's first look at the *tumor infiltration process*.

You Will Learn about Tumor Poisons that Disrupt Cancer Cell Division

As you work to get your diet under control — to deprive cancer of its sixteen-times sugar lifeline — simultaneously, you should introduce infiltration tactics to disrupt cancer's cell division rates. These tactics include the following:

CBD Oil with Frankincense, Saffron & Baking Soda

Cancer cells, part of the host body, are often difficult to detect; technically, they are host cells gone astray, not outside foreign invaders. You can help the immune system identify these insiders as "bad guy" targets. The CBD oil attaches to tumor cell wall receptors making the tumor visible to the immune cells so that immune agents attack the now-visible tumor as a foreigner.

Frankincense and cumin seed oils are mixed into the CBD oil as stealth agents designed to infiltrate tumors already clinging to the CBD molecules. Working together, they confound each cancer cell's propensity to divide and arrest the tumor's growth rate thus providing time for the immune cells to whittle down the tumor.

Honey or Maple Syrup Laced with Baking Soda

Foods that help with alkalinity are discussed in the book's diet section. Here we use food— honey and maple syrup—to trick cancer, a Trojan horse tactic. Baking soda is extremely alkaline and can be added to either honey or maple syrup, then heated up so that the baking soda molecules attach to the honey or maple sugar molecules. Once you ingest the combined mixture, the sugar-starved cancer tumors vigorously ingest the sugar (similar to a PET Scan application); the tumors inadvertently also ingest high concentrates of alkaline-based baking soda in the process, a substance they detest. This formula is described in the book.

Green Tea Supplements

The book explains that cancer cell receptors only listen for "divide" signals broadcast by your hormonal system; "die" signals are not heard. To address this problem, cancer ENOX2 receptors need to be "plugged" to prevent divide signals from reaching the cancer cell's nucleus—don't let cancer hear anything! (We describe ENOX2 receptors later.)

A compound in green tea fits nicely in the cancer cell's ENOX2 hormone receptor "antenna," thereby blocking incoming stimulus.

You Will Learn about Toxins and Oxidative Stress and How these Enable Cancer Occurrences and Growth

Your internal chemistry is a finely tuned system. You need to eliminate foreign elements for your body to operate at optimal levels. Once your chemistry is compromised, your cells become vulnerable to oxygen (burning) and viral attack. Your diet needs to supply your cells with a steady supply of antioxidants to protect them from being chemically compromised. The diet and supplement chapters of the book cover this.

You Will Learn how to Empower Your Immune System to Aggressively Attack Your Tumors

Now that we have starved and then tricked the cancer tumors with self-inflicted poisons and hormonal plugs, it is time for the coup de grâce, the *execution* of these diminished cells. The executioners comprise various immune system cells all described in detail within the body of this book. The supplements described below stimulate and feed these various immune cells.

Red Reishi Mushroom Extract–The Stimulant

This extract comes from Red Reishi mushrooms originally found in Japan. The organic molecules from the mushroom "heal" imbalances throughout the body allowing, for example, the liver to operate without stress and constraints. Compounds in Red Reishi also invigorate immune cells making them more vigilant in attacking tumors.

Beta-Glucan – Immune Cell Vitamins

Beta-glucans are organic molecules found in many plants and are essential vitamins for immune cells. If your diet alone does not yield sufficient levels of glucans, then the immune cells become sluggish. On the other hand, if you have too much beta-glucan in your bloodstream, kidney and liver functions simply wash it out. Hence, especially as you age, it behooves you to take a daily dose of glucans just as you would take vitamin C. Both vitamins are water soluble and flushed out of your system daily, thus requiring replenishment. Glucans are food for immune cells, so feed them!

Resveratrol Opening Capillaries

Resveratrol pills come from red grape skins. These organic molecules relax the circulatory pathways, lowering stress on the heart and enabling better transport of oxygen, nutrients, and immune cells throughout the body. Avoid gridlock, take resveratrol.

You Will Learn about Iodine and Dense Breast Tissue

Cancer is triggered when cells divide incorrectly. This occurs when cells, weakened by carcinogens and oxidative stress, allow infection by viruses. Because a vast amount of cell division occurs in the breast tissue during menstrual cycles, breast tissue has special provisions to combat viruses that are lurking about looking for vulnerable cells.

First, breast organs use iodine — an antiseptic — fed from the thyroid gland. Women with thyroid issues probably lack sufficient iodine levels. Other naturally-based anti-viral supplements will also be described.

Second, due to repeated, monthly cell division and cell death in the breast tissue, scar deposits build up causing a dense breast tissue condition, impeding nutrient, oxygen, and immune support to the breasts.

Dense breast conditions quadruple your chances of getting cancer. Younger woman under thirty have enzymes that remove scar tissue. Older woman over thirty no longer generate these enzymes and need to use primrose oil and the scar-busting serraflazyme supplement to avert dense tissue buildup.

You Will Learn how to Boost Oxygen and Energy Levels in Your Body

As you age, the amount of oxygen reaching your cells, and the amount of energy produced by those cells declines making them susceptible to disease while also impeding the immune system in fighting disease. You must restore oxygen and energy to healthier levels when confronting cancer, and this book offers numerous ways to achieve this.

Sleep — You Will Learn how the Nervous System Regulates Sleep and why Sleep Is Key to Recovery

Basically, a daytime nervous system dominates while you are awake and a nighttime nervous system takes over during sleep when the healing functions operate. You must foster these systems to keep them on track or else healing functions are compromised.

You Will Learn about Statistics

When engaged with medical writing, you must understand the ways of statistics so as NOT to misinterpret conclusions. For example, take the use of percentages. Percentages can naturally mislead you as follows: The overall chance of developing breast cancer is 1 in 8, or approximately 12%. Studies show that hormonal contraceptives increase your risk by 7%. This 7% is not additive, which together would bring your risk to 19%. It refers to 7% of 12%, which comes to 1%. Your risk of developing breast cancer if you used hormonal contraceptives is 13% — higher than normal (12%), but only marginally.

You Will Learn of the Various Breast Medical Conditions and the Types of Breast Cancers, plus You Will Ponder the Incubation Time Cancer Takes to Develop before It's Detected

It can take anywhere from eight to fifteen years for cancer to become visible. The self-healing plan proposed in this book seeks to a) slow this rate, or better, b) reverse the rate, shrinking budding colonies, or best, c) eliminate colonies altogether. All three results are welcome.

Okay, that's a high-level look at what's to come inside the book. **But you need to read the actual journal to cross the finish line.** So become a student! Read the book's journal details and watch the videos before signing up for invasive medical procedures that ignore these considerations. Some cancer doctors will dismiss all of this as nonsense; others will

---

patronize you, saying, "Well...it can't hurt," and some will say they welcome naturopath assistance "to ease the effect" of radiation and chemotherapy. But none will encourage you to try an all-out naturopath plan for ten to twelve weeks to see if it shrinks your tumors, thereby avoiding radiation, chemotherapy, and surgery altogether. And keep in mind the following:

You will not eliminate your cancer by ingesting the abbreviated list of supplements previously described; you eliminate cancer by totally immersing yourself intellectually into understanding your personal biological system, understanding how it works, and taking many, many small steps that collectively tip the scales against the renegade cancer cells.

You are not a victim of cancer. Cancer is simply a malfunction within you and needs to be arrested within; hence, you need to know the details of what is going on inside your body. No handwringing allowed!

Alternatively, you can do the opposite, that is, outsource the problem to radiologists, oncologists, and surgeons who kill cancer cells via physical intervention with noted collateral and permanent damage and without any improvement of the body's defensive systems going forward.

You should not stumble into decisions on how to eliminate your cancer. You should know all you can, hence this book, which describes some of the know-how coming from the naturopathic side of the equation.

Decide for yourself.

Empower yourself.

But before getting into the book proper, please consider other matters you should understand about the world of traditional cancer treatment. You will be up against it, so you need to know about it.

The Medical–Intervention Complex

Admittedly, "*Defeating Breast Cancer*" recommends a disciplined plan dealing with sugars, toxins, and energy levels, but one we believe to be far superior to the short-term "survival statistics" proffered by cancer researchers, pharmaceutical manufacturers, surgeons, radiologists, and oncologists. These medical interventionists propose surgery, chemotherapy, and radiation as the central options for cure, and they frame success only in terms of improved five-year survival rates.

Conversely, the payoff for pursuing *self-healing* proves immeasurable. Not only will you blunt cancer without assaults on your body but you will also emerge from self-healing in the best condition imaginable, the best of your life—at an ideal weight, with full energy, and with optimal skin and muscle tone for your age. You will have started "sick" and ended up as the saying goes, "better than ever," with time itself no longer an eminent threat, and you, yourself, in control. *You* monitor your status, and *you* call the shots. Along the way, as you monitor the shrinking of your cancer with periodic assessments, reassured that self-healing works for you, your personal health status will prove to be the only statistic that truly matters, not the statistics of others. Yet, due to the plan's complexity, the need to overcome food addictions, and the persistent time commitment, self-healing may not work for everyone. It requires you to assume the role of an action hero fighting for your own results. Standard medicine keeps you passive all the while weakening your body and psyche with surgical invasions and needle insertions and weakening every cell in your body with radiation and drug bombardments that ignore the root cause of your condition. However, some people, even after reading *Defeating Breast Cancer* and accepting all or most of it, will find self-healing too demanding and instead opt for these brutal surgery/radiation/chemo solutions, hoping to gain whatever potential for an extended life these plans offer.

"At my age," you might reason, "standard medicine (such as it is) offers the only bet I can tolerate, anyway." By reading *Defeating Breast Cancer*, you will discover which bet suits your orientation: brutal medical intervention or extended personal discipline.

Nope, there's no "Get Out of Jail Free" card in *this* game. Most of the women we have spoken to claim that they have the discipline to implement the plan... and we believe most do, with the majority of readers using this book as a cancer prevention guide. But don't think that self-healing only works for early-stage cancer; the leverage also applies to later stages of the disease, although, admittedly, at some point, nothing can save you once the disease overwhelms your body.

But be mindful. You *can* elect to do both self-healing *and* medical intervention. Even if you go with medical intervention, you can still adopt self-healing before and after medical intervention to test and strengthen your body.

Consider this: Before reaching the point of no return, over expanded cancer colonies depend completely upon the fixed, moment-by-moment nutritional resources the bloodstream offers and are therefore more easily deprived through dietary measures. And once diet deprives cancer cells and they become increasingly impotent, the billions of *empowered* immune system cells the body musters every second can tip the scales, bringing death and destruction to the weakened colony day and night. More developed cancer may take longer to wear down, but it still remains vulnerable.

And do not forget the *infiltration* tactics where things cancer tumors hate can directly assail them without hurting the body—things such as heat, common baking soda, oxygen, green tea, saffron, CBD oil, and even frankincense (the specifics are described in detail within the book). Until now, your cancer resided on Easy Street, never facing all three frontal assaults. You never deprived it of sugar, even for a moment; your immune system never launched an all-out attack, and certainly natural poisons never infiltrated it making *it* feel sick every second of its existence. Through *zero-sugar, empowered immune defenses,* and various *tumor infiltration tactics,* the plan turns your body into a medical powerhouse able to impinge both current and future rogue cancer cells.

Defeating Breast Cancer also details specific theories of what causes a normal cell to turn cancerous. Every serious person ponders, "What is the actual cause?" So, why not explore the possibilities?

We propose that viruses, "ninja-like" parasites, infiltrate normal but enfeebled cells and take them over during cell division at the DNA level, flipping genetic switches, turning cells cancerous. Some dismiss this viral explanation as not proven. They instead believe that *risk factors,* such as cigarette toxins and alcohol, cause *spontaneous genetic mutations* that turn healthy cells into cancer during *cell division,* yet they provide no further details on how such "spontaneity" takes place so consistently from person to person. At any rate, prepare yourself to contemplate the topic on the root cause of cancer to gain a deeper look into the world of cellular biology at the conceptual level.

Most cancer doctors will not initiate a discussion of biological subjects as they do not for a minute believe that you can or should understand them. Rather than engaging you with cause-and-effect concepts, cancer doctors merely offer patients game-show-like "Door #1" and "Door #2" treatment options in a most perfunctory manner, simply citing survival rates. Doctors believe they embody "real science," employing the best techniques and procedures possible. Everything else remains dangerous fantasy proposed by wishful amateurs with no data to hang their hopes on. Nevertheless, and without capitulating to their single-mindedness, you can always employ doctors when conditions merit their expertise; but again, *you* call the shots.

Most doctors fall victim to the data-driven doctrines molded at the medical schools of their youth, all of which deal with the statistical outcome of intervention methods such as chemo, radiation, and surgery. And, once in practice, they stay on this track reinforced by the conformist thinking of their esteemed colleagues, so much so that they cannot dare to proffer non-intervention, non-statistical self-healing possibilities. And thus, women with breast cancer are effectively denied this choice.

Also, no matter how cancer doctors feel personally regarding alternative cures, they have no choice but to keep quiet as they risk litigation if, for example, they recommend self-healing and the patient only follows it halfheartedly and fails. Additionally, the American Medical Association discredits any doctor who strays from the medical profession's sanctioned treatments.

Insurance companies drive the market paying only for treatments sanctioned by mysterious medical-bishops who have the final say in how much society will pay—and for what. These vast, powerful economic forces have nothing to do with your best interests, and we are sorry to say, you must keep the medical industry's intellectual prejudices and economic motivations top-of-mind at all times when interacting with a "medical professional." But before you tangle with the entire "medical–intervention complex," we suggest you first be fully armed with the know-how presented in *Defeating Breast Cancer*"—or otherwise face being overwhelmed.

For the record, I do not oppose surgery, chemotherapy, or radiation per se and would have willingly employed these if my self-healing attempt did not reverse or at least arrest my condition in the three-month time frame we set to try all of this.

After reading *Defeating Breast Cancer*, you will enjoy far superior conversations with any doctor, nutritionist, or specialist you consult regarding causes and cures. And if what they claim does not ring true, you can continue on your own way without fear.

Enough said. Now let's get to the good news: The results!

In one year's time, my cancer tumors were no longer visible on the mammogram, and I literally sparkled with energy and vitality. We next entered our "trust, but verify" years of watching my health closely using semi-annual 3D sonograms to examine my breast and lymph tissue.

We wrote *Defeating Breast Cancer* in story form so that the reader could discover and accumulate *know-how and courage* the way we did, one nugget at a time. Regardless of your cancer tumor type, start with *Defeating Breast Cancer* as the basis for obtaining a general, plain-speaking understanding of the immune system, digestion, toxicity, acidic-versus-alkaline blood, free radicals, energy, oxygen, cellular architecture, cell receptors, hormonal signaling, the nervous system and sleep, and the cause and treatment of cancer. Some advisors suggested that we cut certain sections of the book they deemed too detailed for the average reader, such as free radical biochemical chain reactions, or the separate digestion paths of sugars and fats, or the section on extrapolating the properties of energy, or the section on the role of individual immune system cells, and so on. They proposed we write a book simply listing the cancer-fighting rules one should follow and be done with it.

Joe and I rejected this *For Dummies* approach because most of the people who we talked to while writing this book wanted to know the *whys, hows, and whats* behind the step-by-step procedures in a cancer-cure rulebook. Plus, we include the writings of many medical researchers to support the details, but we present them in context to facilitate their understanding by laypeople. Medically, the plan worked, and by exploring the science and the theories behind it, you, too get to weigh in with your own thoughts on the complete set of causes and effects proposed herein.

The one thing we can assure you of is this: Understanding the body's biochemical/energy design will give you the confidence you need to fend off cancer yourself. Indeed, knowledge *is* power.

By the way, we would not have documented *Defeating Breast Cancer* except for the encouragement—a direct command actually—from our second daughter, Tara, then age nineteen, who insisted, "You'd better start writing it all down… before you forget it."

We brushed Tara's suggestion aside, saying, "No one wants someone else telling them how to do things."

Her response? "Well, if you reach just one woman and you help her, isn't that worth the effort?"

I hope you are that woman.

Laura Patrina,
2019

The Journal

By Joe Patrina

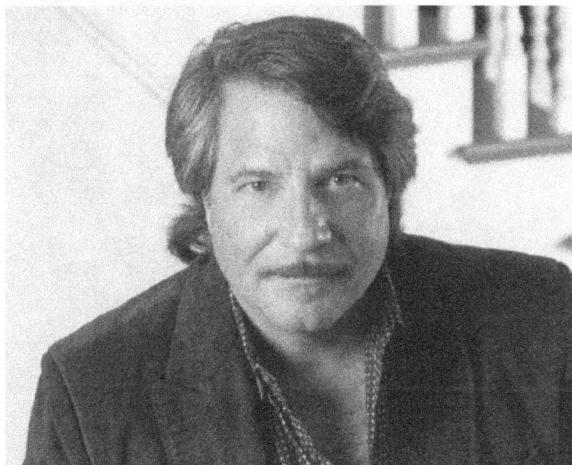

Part I

Meeting Cancer

Chapter 1

The Phone Call

*L*aura got the phone call. She was diagnosed with Stage 1A breast cancer. For some reason, she waited all day to tell me. The mammogram reveals two tumors in her right breast: a larger, nine-millimeter node (the size of a pencil eraser) at three o'clock, and a smaller, four-millimeter node below it, at around five o'clock. The relatively small tumor sizes draw the Stage 1 rating (Stages 1-4 are described below). Discovered by way of mammogram and verified a few days later by a powerful sonogram, both tumors are biopsied with a needle designed to clip a piece of flesh so that the local pathology lab can determine the specific tumor cell type. The biopsy procedure also places two tiny titanium markers inside of the breast next to the tumor nodes to easily locate them in the future.

I felt uneasy about the biopsy as I thought for certain the needle procedure would break off many tumor cells allowing them to spread. At the time, I said nothing.

There are three main types of breast cancer cells with Laura's the most common. Referred to as estrogen-sensitive breast cancer, this cell type is found in 70 percent of breast cancer cases. Laura gets a second phone call from her gynecologist when the pathology department at Hartford Hospital in Connecticut positively identified the cancer cell type as estrogen sensitive. The hospital keeps the biopsied tissue on file at the lab in the event other doctors want to examine it.

The Different Types of Breast Cancer:

- *Estrogen or Progesterone Sensitive*: Of all breast cancers, 70 percent grow in response to the hormone estrogen and about 65 percent of these also grow in response to the hormone progesterone. These hormones, which fluctuate in intensity with the menstrual cycle, do not cause the cancer; they instead urge the cancer to multiply, that is, to grow in response on a *cyclical* basis (more on this later).

- *HER2 Positive:* Of all breast cancers, 20 percent are HER2 positive where having too many copies of the HER2 gene in your DNA causes the production of high levels of the HER2 protein inside the cell. Similar to estrogen (described above), the HER2 proteins tell cells to grow and divide, but because HER2 is always present, that is, *noncyclical*, HER2 breast cancer often proves more aggressive.

- *Triple Negative*: An extremely aggressive form of breast cancer, unrelated to 1) estrogen, 2) progesterone, or 3) HER2 factors, hence the Triple Negative moniker. Approximately 10 percent of breast cancer cases are Triple Negative, and they are the worst for reasons I could not uncover (maybe the cancer profession only knows what this cancer is *not*—it is *not* estrogen, progesterone, or HER2 driven, and hence it is treated with different, *nonreceptor*-based, chemotherapies).

A few days later, Laura and I meet with a recommended breast cancer surgeon at Hartford Hospital who, with a magic marker, draws us a sketch of a human breast on the sheet of paper covering the examination table. He lays out but two options: 1) a *lumpectomy*, cut out the tumors and also cut out a few related lymph nodes as well, and then radiate both the right breast and the remaining right armpit lymph nodes for fifty days; or option 2) a full mastectomy of the right breast and armpit lymph nodes with no radiation required (because there's nothing left to radiate).

I stand aghast at this whole nonchalant presentation.

The lymph nodes, by the way, are removed in case some of the cancer tumor cells have drifted from the tumor to a nearby lymph gland via the lymphatic system. The possibility that escaped cancer cells sat trapped in the three or four breast-drainage lymph nodes was cited as a serious concern.

I interject that I oppose removing the armpit lymph nodes as this impinges the lymphatic pathway out of the arm and chest cavity for the ongoing needs of the lymphatic vessels. In addition, loss of nodes can lead to swollen arms and other permanent side effects because the surgery can cause scarring and blockage of the lymph vessels.

The *lymphatic system* is a separate system from the blood system with its own vessels that, among other jobs, drain dying cells and transport immune cells (more on this later).

The surgeon brushes off my worries about surgically removed lymph nodes and goes on to present survival statistics for his two recommended procedural options — lumpectomy and full mastectomy — confidently proclaiming the improved life expectancy rate of each out to five years.

I know a few women sixty to eighty-plus years old who have survived breast cancer. Ultimately, they had unwittingly chosen both alternatives. The problem? Over the long term, it always ended up in a double mastectomy:

The first breast cancer occurrence would be treated by lumpectomy and radiation and the patient would be good for a number of years.

Then cancer would develop in the second breast in, say, year eight, again treated by lumpectomy and radiation.

Then, by year fourteen, cancer occurred in the original breast again, this time requiring a mastectomy as you cannot use radiation a second time.

Finally, cancer occurred again in the second breast, too, leading to the final double mastectomy.

Even after a double mastectomy where there is no breast tissue left, the cancer still can resurface by metastasizing into a different cell type such as lung or bone cancer.

In the cases that I am aware of, the root cause of the cancer was never discussed let alone treated, so the cancer — probably never completely eradicated — just kept coming back. Laura, at fifty years old and the mother of four, wanted to live another thirty to forty years if possible, and all of this talk about five-year survival horizons flabbergasted and frightened us. Besides bringing up gruesome long-term survivor stories like these, I also tell the doctor that I had direct experience with cancer because of the death of my first wife some thirty years ago. He grimaces knowing what was to come, but I tell the story anyway.

In the late 1980s, my first wife, Janna, succumbed to Hodgkin's lymphoma (a blood cancer) after an eleven-year fight. We had embraced the whole chemo/radiation/surgery program to the hilt at places like Sloan Kettering and Mount Sinai in New York City until the end when doctors finally said she had but one week to live.

Only then did I muster the guts to start her on the macrobiotic cancer diet (a Japanese vegetarian diet) I had been studying for a year. The day I brought her home, I hired two cooks to prepare the macrobiotic vegetarian-based meals. A week later she was stable. A month later, she was out of her wheelchair going for walks. Two months later, she was taking cabs to cooking school learning how to prepare the dishes. For a while, she and I glowed with newfound health. I knew that her tumors were still holding on for dear life, but nevertheless they were shrinking, passive, and no longer causing physical trauma.

And then, after a Thanksgiving holiday where Janna endured everyone else's festivities while she ate only vegetables, I returned home from work to find her chain-smoking cigarettes saying that her fight days were over. Janna died six months later of pneumonia, a year more than promised by her cancer doctors.

Thirty years later, with Laura, my second wife, I hold no desire to repeat the delayed blunders of the past and want to consider the diet and holistic tract from the get-go with a woman whom I consider perfect both physically and psychologically. With Laura, a black-belt karate trainer, I know that her mind/body strength can defeat cancer if we get her going on all fronts: toxin cleansing, nutrition optimization, immune system boosting, oxygen enhancement, energy balancing, ongoing exercise, stress elimination, and so on, and, hopefully, by also implementing innovative tactics, referred to as *infiltration*, that would really hurt cancer cells, my favorite part of the plan.

I certainly do not want to submit to aggressive medical intervention that weakens Laura under the auspices of saving her. Laura possibly might accept the lumpectomy without cutting out the lymph nodes, but months of radiation grates against her survival instinct and she makes that abundantly clear. Instead, the day she learns of her diagnosis, Laura cuts out all sugars, white carbohydrates, wine, dairy, and so on. Cancer cells need many times the amount of glucose sugar as do normal cells, so by going cold turkey with sugar, you cut off the cancer's food supply that very day. Let's call it "zero tolerance."

Laura, "The Lioness," suddenly began the prowl! But we stood only at the beginning of a comprehensive plan to stymie the cancer.

I tell all of this to the crestfallen surgeon. And so, before scheduling a surgical procedure for the next week (as the surgeon had suggested at the top of the meeting), I say that we want to take a breath or two and think this through. For one, we want to meet with a BRCA specialist to determine if Laura is genetically predisposed to breast cancer. The surgeon's office finds a BRCA analyst at the hospital for us to meet in a few days' time, and we rescheduled to meet with the surgeon a second time a week later. But upon breaking up the meeting, the surgeon cautions me by saying that Laura's nine-millimeter tumor holds over a billion cancer cells and the four-millimeter tumor around 500 million. In addition, many cancer cells and microtumors likely lurk as well, too small to be detected.

These gigantic numbers get to us. We leave feeling wobbly and in trouble. That night, I research the basics to create ballast for our little boat, and I find answers for these questions:

What Are the General Medical Issues Concerning the Breasts?

These are the breast conditions as cited on the American Medical Association (AMA) website:

Fibroadenomas are fibrous, *benign* (noncancerous) growths in breast tissue. These growths are solid, usually painless lumps that are not attached to any structures in the breast. A fibroadenoma is usually removed surgically using a local anesthetic.

A cyst is a fluid-filled sac. The cause of breast cysts is unknown. In the vast majority of cases, cysts are not harmful although they may cause pain. Cysts disappear sometimes by themselves, or your doctor may draw out the fluid with a needle. (Recently, women told me that some doctors still recommend mastectomies for cyst conditions.)

A breast abscess is a collection of pus resulting from an infection. Symptoms may include tenderness and inflammation. Antibiotics are prescribed to treat the infection, and your doctor may drain the pus.

Fibrocystic breast disease is a common condition characterized by an increase in the fibrous and glandular tissues in the breasts, which results in small, nodular cysts, noncancerous lumpiness, and tenderness. Although called a "disease," this condition is *not* a disease. There is no specific treatment for fibrocystic disease. (Note: I will suggest a treatment in chapter 18.)

*A **tumor*** that is precancerous or cancerous usually shows up as a white area on a mammogram even before it can be felt. In cases where the tumor is cancerous, it may appear as a white area with radiating arms. A cancerous tumor may have no symptoms or may cause swelling, tenderness, discharge from the nipple or indentation of the nipple, or a dimpled appearance in the skin over the tumor. A breast biopsy is helpful in determining whether a mass is cancerous.

I also get a handle on the official stages of breast cancer as follows:

Stage 1A — Small tumors less than 2 cm growing in the original place the cancer developed (called "in situ").

Stage 1B — Evidence that cancer cells have spread to the lymph nodes in the armpit.

Stage 2A — The tumor has grown to 2-5 cm or three lymph nodes are infected.

Stage 2B — The tumor has grown larger than 5 cm or four lymph nodes are infected.

Stage 3 — Stage 3 breast cancer has extended beyond the immediate region of the tumor and may have invaded nearby lymph nodes and muscle.

Stage 4 — Stage 4 breast cancer has spread to distant organs of the body.

Next, I glean a basic understanding of the internal battlefield once cancer takes root:

How Does Cancer Spread?

Newly infected cells, now cancerous, are usually killed off by the immune system.

Normal cells turning cancerous become more common as you ages and as your general health deteriorates.

If the immune system falls behind, unchecked cancer cells form colonies (tumors).

Tumors feed off of the body's blood system, capillaries at first, but then seek to envelope larger blood vessels to increase the nutrients they take in and their growth rate. With a supply of sustained nutrients, tumors can grow to many billions of cells in size.

After digesting all of the above until 5 a.m., I am ready to brief Laura who, once awake, is pretty pissed off that the doctors had not briefed us first. Each night I pursued further research, attempting to connect all sorts of dots, my brain exhausted. I wanted to acquire an informed and measured position in advance of our next meeting with the breast surgeon, but this challenge proved daunting.

Chapter 2

Getting Help

A week—seven days—is a lot of time in one sense but no time whatsoever when you hold the dread of billions of cancer cells running loose.

As I said in the previous chapter, after first leaving the surgeon's office, I knew I would hop on the Internet and go into both cyber and book research mode six to ten hours per day, digging into the world of breast cancer to find plans for each of the previously mentioned offensive fronts: diet, immune system, cleanses, and so on. But with our heads swimming, Laura and I needed to meet with trusted advisors to fully sort things out before our next meeting with the surgeon.

The first stop? Our local naturopath doctor, Cheryl Vincent. We met with her that very day right after the kick-off meeting with the surgeon. This holistic doctor had treated many members of my family from prescribing nutritional supplements, identifying allergies, healing sprains (using photon-light therapy) to correcting chiropractic conditions.

I consider her an encyclopedia of alternative medicine. From this meeting emerged three initiatives:

First, Laura would start a fourteen-day cleansing diet that included enzymes to relax her organs and fat cells into releasing deeply stored toxins and excess triglycerides.

Second, we would go to Boston to meet with a thermography analyst who would identify points of trauma in Laura's body.

Third, the holistic doctor drew a blood sample and sent it to a lab to determine the absorption level of forty or so vitamins and minerals deep inside Laura's white blood cells. The findings from the lab would dictate the nutritional supplements needed.

The BRCA Meeting

Coming up next ahead of the thermography trip to Boston is another trip to Hartford Hospital to meet with the BRCA specialist.

The American Cancer Society introduces BRCA as follows:

"BRCA1 and BRCA2 are human genes that produce tumor suppressor proteins. These proteins help repair damaged DNA, and therefore play a role in ensuring the stability of the cell's genetic material. When either of these genes is *mutated*, or altered, such that its protein product is not made or does not function correctly, DNA damage may not be repaired properly. As a result, cells are more likely to develop additional genetic alterations that can lead to cancer."

In other words, the BRCA genetic trait itself does not "cause" cancer. Instead, if these genes are weakened, they are unable to repair damaged DNA thereby allowing free radical and viral attacks on cells to succeed. (I assume Angelina Jolie understood this distinction when electing a double mastectomy.)

We arrive at the office of the BRCA specialist expecting to have another blood test drawn and sent to the genetics lab for evaluation. Instead, Laura fills out a questionnaire about her family background, and the analyst enters these facts into a computer.

"Tada." The software package concludes that Laura's collective family and ethnic backgrounds make Laura not suitable for BRCA testing. Apparently, we are neither getting a blood test nor even human expertise to weigh in on the matter at hand. It takes me a while to decipher that a summary judgment was just delivered by a twenty-eight-year-old data input clerk. We figure that being in a life-and-death cancer situation, a definitive BRCA analysis report would be a good thing and that a blood test would make perfect sense.

After mildly interrogating the analyst, I discover her to be an insurance company filter. In other words, if your probability for BRCA is low, then insurance is not required to cover the $5,000 tab for BRCA testing! The filter worked. The twenty-something clerk says that if we want to, we can pay the 5 Gs ourselves, out-of-pocket. I said we would think about it... and we left.

That this Hartford Hospital service was a filter for the insurance companies was an eye-opener. The silver lining to this mostly wasted day? The questionnaire told Laura that she possessed a low probability of BRCA deficiency. But as you might guess, I hate probability statistics when we can obtain clear data. I would reconsider BRCA testing down the road once we lined up the other ducks. (BTW, we paid for this ridiculous meeting with our credit card, out-of-pocket.)

The Thermography Meeting

Two days later, we witnessed the clever world of thermography in action. The basis of this test holds that traumatized areas of the body retain concentrations of warm blood, as blood delivers platelets, T-cells, killer cells, and stem cells to the area in trouble. We can identify these areas of warm blood concentration by placing the body as a whole in a cold environment where blood, in general, rushes to the body's core to protect the organs with only the traumatized spots left still holding significant levels of warm blood. *Normal areas become cool, but traumatized areas remain warm.*

It was a two-and-one-half-hour drive from Connecticut to the outskirts of Boston, but we eventually found the building. The waiting room held books on diet that I perused. I remained skeptical about what would come next even though I understood the straightforward premise of the whole thermography program.

The analyst, Jackie Bell, proved a veteran in her field of expertise, competent and articulate. She first measured one hundred body surface temperature points on Laura's head, neck, and torso in a comfortable temperature setting. Once these readings registered, she cooled the room and activated fans causing body chills. The analyst remeasured the one hundred temperature points and thus identified three points of trauma: (1) *in the jaw, at tooth numbers 3 and 4; (2) in the valve between the small and large intestine; and (3) in the thyroid gland.*

With these findings, things grew very interesting…

First, Laura's only lifetime dental issues comprised an extracted tooth number 3 eight years before and a root canal on tooth number 4 one year before.

Second, a kinesiologist, Doctor Karpenko (a *kinesiologist* measures energy flow blockages in the body), had recently identified a weakness in Laura's small/large intestine valve area (she complained of bloating and pain) and had given Laura exercises to strengthen the area. These exercises greatly improved her condition, yet some sensation remained.

Third, Laura's thyroid condition had been treated with T3/T4 supplements for around six years as her thyroid gland was apparently failing to deliver these needed hormones.

More compelling was that the *energy meridian* (the life force channel), which went through the cancerous tumors on Laura's right breast, started at the traumatized teeth numbers 3 and 4 and ran to the traumatized intestinal valve — *point-to-point*. An immediate possibility was that the level of life force energy flowing down the meridian through the affected breast area was chaotic, preventing breast cells and local immune cells from getting the energy reinforcement (stimulus) needed to fight off disease. In addition to these findings, the thermography analyst gave me the name of a cancer clinic in Mexico that she urged us to consider.

Back home the next day, we report the events to Doctor Vincent, our naturopath, and based upon the findings, she next recommends a biological dentist who can weigh in on the role of the traumatized teeth. We make an appointment to meet this dentist and make a reciprocal appointment with a gastroenterologist to get a colonoscopy performed on Laura to examine her intestinal connecting valve with the small intestine. We made these appointments two weeks out, so for now, Laura did the fourteen-day cleanse our naturopath recommended, and we put the kinesiologist, whom we had initially consulted for abdomenal pain, in charge of balancing Laura's overall energy levels using chiropractic and acupuncture means on a weekly basis.

In the meantime, I looked into the Mexican clinic.

Mexico

I find the Mexican doctor's *Hope4Cancer* website. It offers a heavy-duty, on-site, three-week assault on cancer including the full-cancer diet, body heating (as cancer hates elevated body temperatures), IV injections (such as vitamin C), and the centerpiece: *photon/sonic oxygen activation therapy.* In this therapy, the patient ingests a compound that only the cancer cells absorb. When subjected to certain light and sound frequencies, this compound chemically unravels releasing huge amounts of oxygen (cancer hates oxygen) into the cancerous tumor. To trigger the oxygen release, the patient lies in a chamber (not unlike a tanning chamber), which directs light and sound waves into the body breaking down the ingested compound inside the cancer cells and releasing oxygen to sicken and kill the cancer.

It sounded like the perfect infiltration strategy.

I searched many websites of prominent research hospitals in America and found that a number of institutions in the United States had, in fact, experimented with photon/sonic oxygen activation. It apparently works yet, for some reason, has not entered mainstream medicine. From what I read, the Mexican doctor gets credit for refining the compound to the point where it only affects the cancer cells.

It took a week, but I finally got to speak to the Mexican doctor whom I found to be very grounded, worldly, and a capable fellow on all accounts. But ultimately, Laura and I passed on his approach (for now), as it weighed heavy in application and long in distance calling for us to be away for almost a month. Since Laura appeared in good health, I first wanted to see what we could do locally and remain centered at home with our four children. Had Laura been a Stage 3-4 case, we may have committed to the three-week program to kick-start the recovery (patients continue with the Mexican program when they return home with some of the approaches described in this book). Also, I would have first wanted more insight into the clinic's results. Certainly, some people have had success there, but is it 1 in 10, 1 in 100, and for what cancers, tumor or blood?

The Second Meeting with the Surgeon

Our seven days passed, and we went back to Hartford to reconvene with the breast surgeon. He appeared to understand our research and motivation and said he did not dismiss any of it, even the Chinese Meridians. But one had to wonder, he postured, if we wanted to live like this, eating limited foods and tending to an elaborate self-help program that held no scientific basis. Or, we could simply do a lumpectomy and get on with life.

We agreed the holistic diet and cleansing approach held no real science, just common sense, but I asserted the surgical approach held no science either, for it merely comprised a body of statistics. True science, I pointed out, explores root causes and effects, *repeatable outcomes*, and not merely probabilities. I further explained our deep-seated fear that in the absence of science, medical intervention pursued neither a root cause nor lasting cure, so we would always be looking over our shoulders. And, as he had admitted, the cancer had been developing for eight to ten years whereby Laura asserted that she had time to try another path.

If we could concoct an organic process of reducing tumor size — proving the body could control the disease — then yes, a lumpectomy (a one-hour procedure) might be warranted, but we could then skip the dreaded six-week radiation follow-up phase. Instead, we would continue with the then-proven holistic measures to kill off the unseen cells left behind after popping out the visible tumors.

Intriguing, yes, the surgeon agreed, but he first wanted us to meet with a radiologist who would make a strong case to do the radiation anyway. His nurse sets up the radiologist meeting, and the surgeon has us sign a document so that another meeting is not needed, just a phone call to schedule a surgery time slot. He *had* proved patient.

Later on, I realized that at no point did anyone ever mention the cost of a lumpectomy plus fifty days of radiation. The cancer world, with ten million insured American patients paying unmentionable amounts of money, year after year, certainly makes for a strange but lucrative "cottage industry."

The Radiologist Visit

A few days later, the radiologist spells out much of the same statistical stuff as had the surgeon. My optic focuses upon gauging the danger of *not* doing the radiation, and with this as my focus, a number of interesting points surface.

First, like the surgeon, the radiologist estimates that the big tumor has been growing for years, maybe as long as eight to ten years (which, as we stated before, corresponded to the infection and extraction of Laura's number 3 tooth and her thyroid issues). Upon her saying this, I wonder about all of the undetectable cancer missed by mammograms and MRIs. I pose that chemotherapy (not her line of treatment) might be a better "mopping up" tactic as it would hit every cancer cell anywhere in the body.

The doctor dismisses this, stating that radiation of the right breast and armpit has better statistical outcomes in these Stage 1 circumstances. I point out that this is only valid in the five-year time horizon. She responds that longer-dated statistics are not available so radiation appears the clearest choice.

The paradox does not dawn on the highly educated doctor who also must have posted some serious SAT and MetCat scores in her day. She just said that the cancer was probably in development for a decade, yet her statistics on success are tied to merely five years. Yes, with radiation, one could have a good five-year result with just the right breast *as other developing cancers elsewhere in the body would only surface later.* I ignore this cockeyed presentation without saying a word.

Finally, I ask if the radiation devices now in use are the same as those employed thirty years back, and she replies, "Basically, yes." Still, Laura and I both take away an important time frame: If it took Laura's tumor that long to get its footing, that is, eight to ten *years or maybe even fifteen years*, then we could go weeks, even months attempting to blunt the tumor's progress before crying "uncle" and signing up for surgery and radiation. We could get a series of sonograms, say, every six weeks, and decide what to do at each checkpoint. With this insight, I, the bold nonpatient, feel the weight of fear quickly receding. Laura, the actual cancer patient, does not feel so confident or clear. But still, she agrees to put on the brakes.

Under the circumstances, fear dominates her psyche at every point and understandably so. A lumpectomy with radiation would silence the fear at least for a few years. The temporary silencing of fear proves the biggest motivator in saying "yes" to standard medical intervention. As the days go by, we talk about this many times, and with so many people saying we should effectively "stop screwing around," the passive surgery and radiation path appears pretty good at many a midnight hour.

The Colonoscopy

As colonoscopy day approaches, Laura says that the ill feelings in her gut have already disappeared after eight weeks of doing the "gut" exercises assigned by the kenisiologist. We go ahead with the exam regardless just to be sure. I admire this gastronomic doctor and his diligence. And so, we are pleased to hear of no visible problems with the large or small intestines or with the connecting valve. While chatting in the recovery room with the doctor about the good findings, I mention the meridian path observations we stumbled upon regarding intestine valve discomfort and traumatized teeth. He dismisses it all as "nonsense." Okay, so he doesn't subscribe to the "find-the- root-cause" approach. Still, his "all clear" report means we are narrowing down the moving parts.

A Laser Treatment Option Surfaces

As I've said before, each night I did research on the Internet. One night, I investigated experimental plans for cancer taking place across the United States. For example, at Columbia-Presbyterian Hospital in Manhattan — near enough to our Connecticut residence no less — I find what appears to be a perfect solution: a facility using a heat laser to directly kill tumor cells with only the incision of a hollow needle affecting the breast. The plan: A heat laser beam flows through the needle's hollow chamber that immediately kills any cells it encounters. A sonogram is used as a guide to target the tumor bit by bit. That morning, I phone the doctor's office at Columbia-Presbyterian and make an appointment for a few weeks out. In the meantime, I arrange to send all of Laura's MRI, ultrasound, and mammogram films to Columbia-Presbyterian and have Hartford Hospital's Pathology Lab mail the biopsy specimen.

We hold great expectations, as a laser expedites the killing of visible cancer tumors to an hour's time, and you could still consider mopping up any hidden cancer cells or colonies by the diet and cleansing approach rather than through radiation or chemotherapy. But candidly, at the time, we lacked confidence that we could kill the tumors on our own. And so, zapping them with a laser beam looked like a pretty good idea. I just couldn't figure out why more professionals did not apply this approach to *all* visible tumor-based cancer cases.

As our appointment stood two weeks away, getting more info about this option would have to wait. But first, our meeting with the biological dentist approached, so next I turned my nighttime research sessions toward understanding the exotic biological dentistry topic, but, even more so, to understand cancer itself—the world of *cells, toxins,* and *viruses* that invade weakened cells.

Chapter 3

The War on Cancer

"*B*ack at the ranch," I pursue my internet research usually working until 3 a.m. each night, sometimes ordering related books on Amazon and reading them cover-to-cover as well. Because I studied cancer in my previous life back in the '70s and '80s during my first wife's ten-year episode, I held a certain curiosity as to what might've changed in the medical world.

Not much, it seemed.

The chemo had grown more "targeted," that is, more devastating to the specific cancer cell type although this approach still poisoned every cell in the body in the attempt to attack this one cell type, and, still, no one discussed root causes. The American Cancer Society's main website page still claims that they do not know what causes cancer, skirting the issue by saying it comprises a collection of factors. They only refer to known risk factors such as cigarette smoking never saying what exactly happens when a good cell turns cancerous.

After fifty years or so of "The War on Cancer," for the medical community to still not offer a definitive cause-and-effect framework seems astonishing. No wonder the whole medical world focuses on cancer *removal* options using the same-old, same-olds: incredibly expensive surgery, poisonous chemotherapy, and debilitating radiation "treatments" rather than nipping cancer in the bud by isolating and removing its germinating enablers at the cellular level.

Let's look at door number three, chemotherapy.

Chemotherapy

Chemotherapy—meaning "curing with drugs"—got its start from experiments with mustard gas stockpiles left over from World War I. Researchers turned the mustard agent (breathed as a burning gas) into a poison that could be infused into the bloodstream. The idea started (and remains) to take advantage of cancer's very active metabolism and rapid cell division rates to absorb poison more aggressively than other cells.

And this is indeed how chemotherapy works; every cell is poisoned with the cancer cells getting it the worst. The poison, though, seriously harms any normal cell that also has fairly high metabolism and cell division rates. These "up-tempo" cells include hair, bone marrow, stomach, and intestine cells. The punishment these innocent cells endure during chemotherapy results in the familiar side effects: hair loss, lowered blood counts, nausea, fatigue, and infections. Not only does chemotherapy weaken all cells but also the chemo drug itself is acidic causing an overall septic condition to settle in throughout the body.

The net result: permanent weakening of the bone marrow, reduced ability to absorb essential nutrients, and emboldened tumors that grow resistant to "chemo" poison — all with nothing accomplished to prevent another bout of cancer to incubate at a future date. With so much negativity surrounding chemotherapy, you might expect a societal pushback of sorts with chemotherapy seen as the modern-day version of bloodletting. Instead, the chemotherapy religion remains stronger than ever. Consider the following taking place in my home state of Connecticut:

On January 3, 2015, Connecticut's newspaper of record, the *Hartford Courant*, reported a story of a seventeen-year-old girl forced by the State Department of Children and Families to accept chemotherapy against her will ("for her own good," they claimed). She suffered from Hodgkins Lymphoma, the same cancer my first wife suffered from. The article explained that the chemo "worked," justifying the whole Orwellian directive.

One final note on chemotherapy: *Postchemotherapy cognitive impairment* (aka "chemo brain") is a condition resulting in changes in memory and fluency affecting many patients treated aggressively with chemo drugs.

What Are the Top-Six Cancer incidents in America?

#1:	Breast Cancer	—	235,000 new cases per year
#2:	Prostate Cancer	—	233,000 new cases per year
#3:	Lung Cancer	—	224,000 new cases per year
#4:	Colon Cancer	—	96,000 new cases per year
#5:	Skin Cancer	—	81,000 new cases per year
#6:	Brain Cancer	—	23,000 new cases per year

That's 800,000 new, top-category cancer cases per year in the United States alone not counting many rare cases. And most telling, the death rate per one thousand due to cancer in America has remained stagnant for decades. The survival rate to five years remains the only improvement. If you are willing to endure surgery, poisoning, and radiation, you might delay death for a short while. And before signing up for treatment, your statistical survival chances are spelled out making the service offering aboveboard and therefore an ethical proposition.

But many things are not pointed out: not a whisper about postchemotherapy cognitive impairment (aka chemo brain), for instance; the steady death rate from cancer over the decades; or the possibilities of self-healing as an alternative.

So much for our "War on Cancer."

Statistics

An important concept to master when getting involved with the medical world is the use of percentages as percentages can naturally mislead you as follows: The overall chance of developing breast cancer is 1 in 8, or approximately 12%. Studies show (see details in the "Loose Ends" chapter) that using contraceptives increase your risk by 7%. This 7% is not additive bringing your risk to 19%. It refers to 7% of 12%, which comes to 1%. Your risk by using hormonal contraceptives is 13% higher, only marginally higher if you did not use contraceptives.

The world of institutionalized medicine is full of percentages; take care.

Tumor Development Time

As mentioned earlier, it can take years for cancer to become visible. The self-healing plan seeks to:

a) slow this rate further; or better,

b) reverse the rate, shrinking budding colonies; or best,

c) eliminate colonies altogether. All three results are welcome.

The following is a tumor growth progression assuming cancer cells double every one hundred days. Recall that tumors need to be in the hundreds of millions before mammograms can detect them.

Day 1:   a single cancer cell is formed

Day 100:   a 2-cancer cell tumor exists

Day 200:   a 4-cancer cell tumor exists

Year 1:   a 10-cancer cell tumor exists

Year 2:   a 50-cancer cell tumor exists

Year 6:   a 1-million cancer cell tumor is well established

Year 8:   a 70-million cancer cell tumor begins to blossom

Year 9:   a 600-million cancer cell tumor becomes visible

Year 10:   a 1+-billion cancer cell tumor becomes very threatening

Part II

Understanding Cancer

Chapter 4

Understanding Cells

It's About the Cells, the Repository of Life

Something turns normal cells cancerous, and later chapter 6 will lay out the virus theory I support. Here in chapter 4, we explore the structure of cellular life as the foundation of more to come. Let's start off with the big picture of life itself — the fundamentals — and then look deeper into cells.

What is life? *It is multidimensional...*

Our Biological Dimension

Human life in its smallest form exists as a cell. Each cell is a *biochemical factory* filled with *molecular and electrical activity*. The cell's DNA and RNA — a vast library of *chemical formula templates* accumulated by each species over generations — direct each cell's molecular activity. An electrically charged *life energy grid* pulsating through the body "commands" cells to operate according to their DNA and RNA chemical formulas. When this *life energy* driver disappears at death,

---

the cellular biochemical processes halt, and we proclaim the entire body "dead" — full stop!

Our Mental Dimension

Whereas your DNA and RNA library holds *inherited biochemical knowledge* that directs and protects the cell, your mental dimension deals with the here and now, directing the body through the nervous system, *somehow* storing *sensory-gleaned experiential knowledge* within the neurons of the brain. Collectively, the brain, a *mental control system*, starts with instinct and further builds a database of acquired knowledge. Some believe that the mind can do even more, claiming that your state of mind can cause — and cure — disease.

Our Consciousness Dimension

Consciousness comprises something more than organized biochemical factories powered by a life energy grid coordinated by a mental control system; for example, zebras possess all of this. *Consciousness*, which, on earth I believe only humans possess, exists where you are aware of your own thinking. Consciousness exists in addition to the biological and mental life dimensions and probably bridges a spiritual world of ideas to us. Knowledge, deciphered and categorized through consciousness, is possibly revealed by the spiritual side; we just tap in.

The limited focus of this book claims that regardless of the source of ideas, our consciousness allows us to envision cures and organize them into effective plans. Consciousness fosters wisdom, hence we are called "sapiens," the Latin word for "wisdom," as in *Homo sapiens*.

The World of Cells

Cells make up the basis of all living things from bacteria to plants to animals. Each cell devours oxygen and nutrients to fuel its biochemical requirements according to the needs set forth by that cell's DNA playbook. The DNA issues orders to the rest of the cell by releasing RNA chemical templates that tell the cell what to do. The released RNA triggers millions of chemical reactions inside and outside of the cell's wall.

These combined DNA and RNA templates are inherited and refined over countless generations toward protecting cells from disease and for governing each cell's "proper" behavior. Moreover, the DNA and RNA templates of each tiny cell work collectively with the other cells of our bodies not unlike a trillion-member symphony orchestra wherein each orchestra member fits exactly into the ensemble knowing its part to play.

Referring to cells as "biological factories" hardly constitutes an exaggeration. Each cell possesses compartments allowing for specialization inside of the cell, for example: the nucleus compartment (the "executive suite"), the mitochondria compartment (the "power station"), and the peroxisome compartment (the "chemistry lab"), and so on. Inside the cell, molecular exchanges called "proton pumps" send enormous amounts of electrical charges around to keep everything running. The cell runs similar to a factory, yet it is *alive* — able to get sick, able to heal itself, able to divide, and able to die.

There are simple cell living things and complex cell living things. Bacteria, for example, exist as simple cell living things. In multi-celled human beings, cells must specialize in their purpose to support this more complex living structure comprising skin, blood, bone, and so on. Humans possess more than one hundred specialized cells (and, by the way, around the same number of cancer types). Estimates put humans housing nearly one hundred trillion cells all pumping away inside of us in super-real time. (I'll use one hundred trillion cells as a reference point.)

Cell Division (*Mitosis*) and Programmed Cell Death (*Apoptosis*)

In addition to the DNA and RNA guided chemistry, which takes place inside the cell, a world of communicative chemistry takes place outside the cell where the cell communicates with the body by further molecular signals.

Certain chemical commanders (*steroids*) direct cells to either divide (*mitosis*) or die (*apoptosis*, from the Greek). Healthy cells will divide or die on command by the body's signals; conversely, cancer cells will ignore the die signals exactly as viruses do (more on this at the end of the book). The balance between dividing cells and dying cells carries paramount importance. If cells only divide and never die, the body would grow indefinitely. Likewise, the command for cells to die must not go overboard if cell populations are to sustain the body in specific locations.

For example, as you age because of such factors as vitamin, mineral, protein, and hormone deficiencies, muscle cells die faster than the creation of their replacements, and the body experiences a slow pattern of muscle loss. Bone weakening provides another common example of the aging factor, though in addition to an imbalance between new and old bone cells, bone weakening also includes changes to the calcium and phosphate content of the bone cell. Age unravels more than one thing.

In complex beings, cells die after a set period of time — skin cells, within weeks; blood cells, in sixty days; and bone cells, years. The rate of cell division must keep pace with this time line of programmed cell death. Uncertainty exists as to which cells will die, although the body apparently quickly chooses "sick" cells because of the molecular signals distressed cells emit (more on cellular "SOSs" later). The test, called "Serum TK," described in the "Living Wisely" chapter, measures the body's overall relationship between dividing and dying cells. High levels of serum TK in adults indicate cancerous activity (runaway division) even if mammograms and other tests cannot "see" the cancer.

Cell Division during Childhood and Menstrual Cycles

Early on, as the body grows during infancy and childhood, most specialized cells divide more rapidly than die (experienced as "growth spurts") until we reach adulthood. Once we achieve maturity, the body somehow maintains the balance between cell division and cell death similar perhaps to a self-balancing gyroscope. At this point, only a few parts of the body still engage in cell divisions that exceed the rate of dying cells. An important example of this — *for the purposes of this book* — comprises the cells of the breast and uterus.

Each month, the body releases quantities of *estrogen*, a hormone-steroid that instructs female sex cells to multiply rapidly in anticipation of pregnancy. If a woman does not become pregnant, the body purges the new cells through menstruation (more on estrogen and menstrual scarring later).

Trauma and Stem Cells

When *trauma* occurs—when cells suffer damage, for example, in an ankle sprain—then the troubled domain broadcasts an alert to attract platelets, T-cells, and stem cells, which rush to the site of the embattled cells to arrest trauma and begin the healing process. But the resolution of trauma takes time. As a reference point, stem cells take up to 60 days to replace a bag of blood donated to the Red Cross and up to 120 days to shore up damaged muscle. Again, these repair activities are not achieved by specialized bone and tissue cells themselves dividing and dying in their normal rhythm but through replacement stem cells moving in. *Stem cells are cells* that are "born" with neutral chromosome settings that mature into specialized cells by copying the settings of the cells they are replacing. (*Chromosome switch settings* that craft specific cellular types are described later.)

Cells not Programmed to Die

Only three types of human cells are not programmed to die: stem cells, heart muscle cells, and neuron cells in the brain.

Stem cells residing in the bone marrow do not live and then die inside the marrow. Instead, stem cells prolifically divide to keep trillions on hand for daily dispersal into the bloodstream by the billions to serve as either specialized replacement cells (for injured body parts) or as new blood cells. However, each time cells divide —whether they are bone marrow cells, skin cells, retina cells, hair cells, and so on—they lose a bit of genetic data much as audio quality deteriorates when copying a recording from tape to tape to tape.

As we age to the point where the cell pool has already divided, that is, has been copied hundreds of times, a meaningful amount of genetic precision erosion results. Thus, weaker body part cells enter play over time. The deterioration of genetic data offers one major reason that age so significantly affects our general level of health and inherently moves us closer to the tipping points of cancer and to natural death. Our cells simply do not know what to do when they are attacked and become vulnerable to outside elements like toxins, viruses, fungi, bacteria, and parasites.

On the other hand, the twenty billion brain neurons that mature by the age of twenty-six — when our frontal lobe stops growing "white matter" — are the only ones we get. No stem cell services create new neurons. Neurons simply fade away as we age; humans lose 1 percent over a lifetime. Because these neuron cells do not divide, their original genetic precision stays intact, and so as long as they are not debased by bad proteins, they prove increasingly effective.

One of the reasons that dementia surfaces in our later years is likely due to rogue proteins that corrode brain and nerve cells and not to a loss of cells. A good protein, called *brain-derived neurotrophic factor* (a growth hormone), helps to repair and grow nerves and create new synapse links among the neurons, but it is unclear if this protein can help generate new neurons to replace dying or damaged neuron cells.

Likewise, the number of heart muscle cells are fixed for life. We die with the same amount of heart cells we were born with. They simply expand as we grow and mature. When heart attacks damage your heart, it remains damaged for life.

I pondered that neither neurons nor heart cells divide; yet brain cancer occurs but not heart cancer. I wrote to the American Cancer Society about this; they acknowledged my e-mail but never responded. Later, I found an article explaining that "binder" gray-and-white matter cells that do divide surround brain neurons, and these binder cells can become cancerous, sometimes because of infection and sometimes from metastasis from other cancerous areas of the body.

With this cellular overview in mind, let's next consider what happens when cells confront toxicity.

Chapter 5

Understanding Toxins

Toxins Cause Acidity and Free Radical Formation

In this chapter, we look at the factors beyond age that weaken cells thus creating a vulnerability to cancer. Four factors thus linked to cancer include toxins, acidity, free radicals, and antioxidants, but they really constitute a single, interrelated phenomenon. It all starts with *toxins*, which include environmental and ingested chemicals plus natural and man-made radiation. These foreign elements transform your healthy biochemistry into a destabilized, inflamed, and polluted environment where bodily fluids become pro-cancer acidic, and renegade molecules called *free radicals* corrode healthy cells. Ugh! Toxins form the common denominator to the entire paradigm, and any attempt to fight cancer that does not include a complete scrubbing of toxins from the body is as useless and ineffectual as washing dishes in dirty water.

Comprehending the vastness of our body chemistry proves a daunting task. Trillions of coordinated, life-sustaining, chemical combinations take place each second in and around the cells, all without causing unwanted molecular by-products that harm the cells. To achieve this level of absolute perfection and balance, body chemistry remains a closed, self-contained, perpetually balanced system, except for one small problem: *Outside chemicals and radiation (the toxins) penetrate the body!* We ingest, inhale, or absorb these foreign substances from the outside, and they trigger a slew of unwanted chemical exchanges resulting in the aforementioned acidity and free radicals.

Let's look at acidity first.

Acidity, Aerobic, and Anaerobic Energy Creation

The body comprises 70 percent salt water, basically the same as the salt concentration in ocean water, both very *alkaline* and able to hold oxygen.

Acidity, in contrast to alkalinity, *squeezes out* oxygen. And so, over the years, as we accumulate acidic chemicals into our cells, oxygen levels decline; the normal cells experience a type of suffocation, and developing cancer cells—which do not use oxygen to generate energy—enjoy an acidic field day all to themselves.

Ninety-nine percent of the time, normal cells use oxygen to burn nutrients (called *aerobic metabolism*)—like burning firewood. Cancer cells (similar to viruses) do not use oxygen to burn nutrients for energy; instead, they rely upon *chemical fermentation* (blending chemicals together, like a whisky still) to create energy for themselves (called *anaerobic metabolism*).

While all cells possess the potential for both aerobic and anaerobic methods, the body remains primarily oxygen based and only uses the anaerobic chemical fermentation method when pushed. Hence, acidic buildup, after years of accumulating toxins in our system, becomes a dangerous state to succumb to as it nudges the body away from oxygen or aerobic methods toward anaerobic reliance. And to make matters worse, there are no clues to indicate this dangerous state is happening.

An interesting way of understanding these aerobic and anaerobic processes is the following: long-distance runners use both processes as the oxygen method alone would not generate sufficient energy to sustain their efforts. The runners' muscle cells, besides devouring oxygen, use uncomfortable anaerobic methods to tap directly into the body's glucose reserves to provide more stamina through chemical mixing (hence, the common practice of devouring carbohydrates before a race). Once the race concludes, the body returns to aerobic methods. A by-product of the racer's anaerobic experience? The creation of lactic acid, which further acidifies the body.

Free Radicals

Environmental and ingested toxic chemicals that cause acidity also interact with other chemicals in the body triggering *free radicals*. Free radicals occur when toxins come in contact with living tissue whereby atomic-level protons and electrons mix and match into new molecular combinations. In this Wild West chemical setting, free radicals form when a molecule's proton and electron counts do not equal one another. A free radical remains standing as a leftover, the molecule stuck without a chair in "Musical Molecules," missing a proton or electron when the chemical music stops.

To correct this proton-electron imbalance, the "radicalized" molecule "robs" elements from nearby healthy cells creating instability in their molecules. These, in turn, steal what they need from the next molecule in the cellular neighborhood and so on. This causes a vast chain reaction in and outside of the cells as electrons and protons are wrested away from stable molecules to make other molecules whole.

The chain reaction progresses like a prairie fire, reaches the cell's DNA and robs its electrons and protons thereby damaging DNA "instruction" genes and gene "switch settings," leaving the cell unable to operate or divide correctly. This damaging of the DNA either leads directly to a cancerous cell division by "spontaneous" mutation (one theory) or it so weakens the cell that viruses can penetrate the DNA and take over through switch settings (the theory proposed in this book).

Either way, cancer can result.

A question: The ability of molecules to carry unbalanced electrical charges is called *ionization*. What I have not been able to determine is why some forms of ionization are damaging and others beneficial. Free radicals, for example, are harmful eating away at the cells. *Electrolytes* (described later) are charged molecules essential for keeping adequate electron supplies within the cells and cause no damage. Hmm.

More on Anaerobic (Nonoxygen) Metabolism

A key insight on how the chain reaction onslaught of free radicals leads to cancer is the effect of free radicals on the tiny *mitochondria* (the cell's energy producers, described in detail in the "Boosting Energy" chapter). Basically, each cell relies upon mitochondria (bacteria-like microbes *living* inside each cell) to create energy for that cell. The mitochondria take in nutrients and burn the nutrients with incoming supplies of oxygen.

If the little buggers suffer damage, or if the cell becomes very destabilized by high acidity or free radical chain reactions, the mitochondria die. When this happens, the cell's whole power station crew shuts down, and the cell remains left to its own devices to survive. The cell achieves survival by switching over to anaerobic metabolism, the backup method (the long-distance runner's auxiliary method) that does not use oxygen. Instead of burning oxygen, the cell ferments chemical combinations that give off heat and electrical charges to create a replacement source of energy.

Anaerobic metabolism processes draw heavily on sugars present in the bloodstream as the main ingredient of their chemical mixing concoction. Cancer cells use this same sugar-based formula to generate energy foregoing oxygen and instead metabolizing sugars, the lifeline of cancer.

And so, though a cell damaged by free radicals may not possess all of the attributes of cancer, such as multiplying freely and metastasizing into new cell forms and so on, the damaged cell contains one key cancerous feature already in operation: *routine anaerobic digestion.*

A full-blown cancer only needs a virus to penetrate its DNA, to propel aberrant RNA orders into the cell, probably by simple switch settings (the theory proposed in this book) and not through mass DNA mutations.

Radiation

Radiation and cancer *correlate* very closely. The probability of cancer increases with the radiation dose you receive, and so theories exist that radiation itself causes DNA mutations turning a normal cell cancerous. This assumes that radiation's cell-damaging method, also a form of ionization (the creation of electron mismatches), can perfectly mutate an entire set of chromosomes and switch settings to work in perfect concert with each other thus behaving as a fundamentally new type of cell. For this to happen, an unimaginable set of coincidences must align. Instead, part of the theory that this book proposes, radiation ionization, like all other carcinogens, causes free radicals to directly reach down to the DNA level (called chromosome "breaks"). This makes radiation just one more way to weaken cells, exposing damaged cells to a viral takeover that infuses the viral "DNA switch" agendas.

Life exposes us to cosmic radiation (from the universe) at all times, but we add to this unavoidable fixed dosage every time we subject ourselves to an x-ray or mammogram. If you also get radiation treatment to kill cancer, then big dosage numbers come into play, which can encourage further occurrences of cancer down the line. As stated earlier, I can imagine circumstances where radiation would offer a reasonable choice to supplement a cancer plan, but it remains a trade-off of survival horizon bets that radiation doctors never discuss.

Oxidative Stress and Antioxidants

Oxygen constitutes one of the important paradoxes of life on earth in its dual role as both friend and foe. We all understand the "friend" part every time we hold our breath and crave oxygen. The "foe" part of the relationship appears less apparent; it is the ability of oxygen to burn things — and not just logs on the fire. Oxygen would burn living matter — our cells — if an oxygen-proof skin did not protect them. For example, an apple's skin protects the apple from the air, but once it is cut open, the internal apple cells become oxidized; the visual evidence is they turn brown and quickly putrefy.

Fortunately, our skin is oxygen proof as is the lung tissue that transports oxygen to the oxygen-proof red blood cells. But like an apple, our internal cells remain vulnerable to "oxidization" (by incoming oxygen). Thankfully, antioxidants come to the rescue.

Antioxidants provide a protective covering that encapsulates each cell's outer membrane, a "chemical skin" of sorts. This covering shields the general membrane from the incoming oxygen allowing specialized membrane receptors to absorb the oxygen in an orderly manner and direct it to its proper destination inside the cell.

Simply speaking, a cell membrane receptor is a molecule sitting on the cell wall that presents a certain puzzle shape that an outside molecule with a reciprocal shape can bind to. All biochemical activities revolve around endless sets of receptor molecules seeking to bind with each other. (The ENOX receptor controlling cell division and cell death will be discussed in detail at the end of the book.)

Antioxidant protective molecules comprise vitamins, such as vitamins A, C, and E, and are provided by the food we eat. Some foods, such as blueberries, contain much higher concentrations of antioxidant support than other foods — hot dogs come to mind as a poor antioxidant. Good antioxidant supplements exist as well. (I discuss the antioxidant food and supplement sources in the "Dietary Supplements" chapter.)

But if you don't have an adequate supply of antioxidants on hand, oxygen will find exposed membranes and oxidize the molecules it encounters. This destructive chemical process, in turn, creates "offspring" free radicals, so now the cell is being burnt while also being chemically destabilized by the chain reactions caused by the free radicals. When we speak about ways to weaken cells, to make them vulnerable to viruses and ultimately to cancer, this "oxidative stress" is on top of the list.

And recall, runaway cellular stress leads to *chronic inflammation* where white blood cells endlessly release repair hormones intended to spur stem cells into healing damaged tissue. But with oxidative stress, there is no role for stem cell healing, yet the oxidatively distressed cell still sends out SOSs. The white blood cells do not know the difference, and inadvertently their repair hormones instead encourage cancer cells to proliferate. Oxidative and carcinogenic stress need to be eliminated to eliminate these open-ended immune system hormonal triggers.

Here's the kicker: As bad as free radicals are, overall, they also serve a purpose. Immune system cells use both oxygen and free radicals as weapons to attack viruses and bacteria lurking in the body. We need certain free radicals, just not every kind, and not too many of those that come in handy. The obvious goal remains to keep the right balance between free radicals and antioxidants, and this requires three steps:

- Detoxify the body of outside chemicals that have built up inside the cells (described in "How to Detoxify"), and
- Consume enough antioxidant foods together with antioxidant supplements to shield against oxidative stress (described in the "Diet" chapter), and
- Stay clear of radiation (a self-evident proposition).

Speaking of radiation, here is a quote from Doctor Blaylot who publishes health advisories:

"An area of medicine that is badly neglected is protecting patients from radiation damage caused by radiological procedures, including CT scans, PET scans, x-rays, mammograms, and injection of radioactive dyes. The danger goes beyond the period of exposure. Damage done by radiation is cumulative and long lasting—which means that each x-ray does more damage, and it builds up over time. When I was practicing neurosurgery, doctors were told by radiologists that CT scans exposed patients to very little radiation. But now we know that a single CT scan can contain radiation that's equal to hundreds of chest x-rays."

An interesting observation follows: Lemons are a great antioxidant food source. Many chefs squeeze lemon juice over cut fruit to keep it from turning brown. Yet fresh-squeezed lemon juice is a great cancer-fighting food for a second reason as well. It is counterintuitive, but citric lemon juice also causes an alkaline response in the body, as chemically the juice reduces the need for the stomach to generate acid.

Triggers in the stomach encountering lemon acid sense that enough acid is in play and do not call upon the stomach glands to produce even more. Reduced stomach acid means that high acidity does not reach the intestines to be absorbed into the bloodstream. Lemons are very good for you, and the famous Mediterranean Diet has plenty of lemons in it.

But before looking at ways to detoxify yourself or to use diet to stabilize your system, we'll next look at how viruses take advantage of polluted and depleted systems, which we claim is the cause of cancer.

Chapter 6

Understanding Viruses

The Seeds of Cancer

We have looked at cells and the toxic factors that weaken cells, so now let's get a feel for the trillions of viruses lying in wait inside and outside our bodies searching for vulnerable cells to live off.

The language below elaborates the *virus theory* that I mentioned earlier, one that I adhere to regarding cancer's root cause at the same time acknowledging that no science per se exists to fully back this theory up. Instead, the viral explanation simply makes sense — at least to me. And if you think I am hanging out on a limb by myself, I found the following statement buried inside The American Cancer Society's website listed under "Viruses" but not under "Cancers."

"Viruses are very small organisms; most can't even be seen with an ordinary microscope. They are made up of a small group

of genes in the form of DNA or RNA surrounded by a protein coating.

Viruses need to enter a living cell and 'hijack' the cell's machinery to reproduce and make more viruses. Some viruses do this by inserting their own DNA (or RNA) into that of the host cell. When the DNA or RNA affects the host cell's genes, it may push the cell toward becoming cancer."

Who knows; the American Cancer Society probably has different camps inside of its own walls each vying for different theories, each neutralizing the other's ability to proclaim their views to the outside world.

So we are on our own. I am on my own!

The World of Viruses

In addition to the vast world of cellular beings, the world of viruses exists as extremely small entities, bigger than atoms, but more than 1/1000 smaller than a cell. Viruses, so stripped down in what they can do, cannot live on their own and therefore must invade and live off cells in parasitic fashion. Virus entities are not preprogrammed to die and do not die until they are destroyed.

For example, chicken pox viruses live inside us for decades and often surface later in life in the form of shingles. Outside of living bodies, viruses can lie dormant for decades in dust and other inert substances, and then brought back to *activity (not life)* when making contact with glucose inside a living being.

Some biologists say that viruses are not true living beings but are instead highly complex chemical systems that become "active" when chemically stimulated by cellular glucose. When a virus penetrates a cell, viral DNA starts to release RNA chemical commands to the cell making the cell do the bidding of the virus. Tactically, viral DNA becomes a reprogramming force (recall HAL, the spaceship's computer in the movie *2001: A Space Odyssey*) that executes a takeover game plan against the cell it has infiltrated.

For an amazing look at viruses in action, check out a vivid animation documentary on the virus and cell battleground produced in England at the following URL:

http://www.dailymotion.com/video/x1f26gz_bbc-our-secret-universe-the-hidden-life-of-the-cell-720p-hdtv_tech

Viruses hate oxygen; oxygen is poison to them. Unlike cells, which oxidize nutrients (remember: burning nutrients like logs on a fire, drafting vast flows of oxygen from the bloodstream), viruses get "free" energy from the host's glucose allowing them to by-pass and effectively hide from oxygen.

By the way, evolutionists believe viruses developed on Earth *before* cellular plants produced oxygen, and hence oxygen remains a "recent" poison for viruses. Still, because symbiotically viruses need cells to survive, I can't fathom the paradoxical assertion by evolutionists that viruses came first...hmm...

Viruses thrive in an acidic bodily environment because acidic plasma chokes off the free oxygen flow coming in from the bloodstream. The bloodstream itself is not acidic — staying always at a Ph level of around 7.4. To maintain this 7.4 level, any acidic substance entering the bloodstream not removed by the kidneys gets parked inside the body's cell chambers and the cells themselves. Over a lifetime large deposits of acid can build up, needing to be purged through detoxification measures.

Viruses multiply by dividing, but when dividing, their DNA (again reminiscent of HAL from the *2001: A Space Odyssey* movie) can metastasize to allow the offspring to better survive obstacles in the immediate environment (for example, to better avoid the body's immune mechanisms, or in the case of HAL" the computer, to be able to outsmart Dave, the astronaut.

Most important, as the American Cancer Society quote explained, when viruses invade cells, the virus ultimately seeks to destroy or switch some of the cells' DNA, substituting its own DNA combo, and effectively "hijacking" the cell itself (this book's viral cancer theory). Viruses usually do not get this far. Sometimes, they penetrate the cells' outer membrane but are killed off inside the cell. Occasionally, they get as far as the inside of the cells' nucleus where they breed a new hive of viruses, perhaps many thousands of them. But occasionally — as you will see shortly with the virus cancer theory — a single virus "hits a home run" and penetrates the cell's DNA messing with genes and gene behavioral switches.

But first a look at the *spontaneous mutation theory*, the theory espoused by most doctors.

Cell Division and the Spontaneous Mutation Theory

We did not discover cell division until the late 1800s. Since then, science determined that the cell goes through multiple staging steps during division. These include preparation steps compressing chromosomes, copy steps splitting chromosomes into sister sets, and reassembly steps building sister sets up to full-fledged DNA and RNA libraries for their own cell plasma entities. Given the chemical and sequencing precision needed to pull this off, the chance of what the doctors refer to as a "spontaneous" mutation happening, a screw-up, always exists along the way.

Mainstream medicine theories out there stubbornly claim cancer happens when a cell's DNA *mutates in a spontaneous manner during cell division*, but this constitutes naïvete in my opinion. Too many thousands of DNA genes and gene–switch molecules — the orchestra members — would have to mutate, all in perfect harmony, for the new cancer cell to live. In other words, and to emphasize this point: *The various thousands of genes and the vast numbers of switch-setting combinations among chromosome strands would require perfect synchronization to keep the emerging cell's biochemical factory operating.* Most true mutations result in cell death as the isolated mutation falls out of step with the vast DNA matrix operating the cell.

The amount of DNA inside a cell can overwhelm your comprehension. Some 20,000 different genes reside within, each gene switched on and off (*expressed*) via millions of molecular switch combinations. These switches are like the brail spindle on a player piano activating piano keys. Certain switch molecules activate sets of genes that determine each cell's assigned role in the body ("you're a skin cell"). Other gene switches happen in real time as the cell spars with the survival circumstances that it encounters — such as hunger, oxygen depletion, toxin and stimulant absorption, hormonal commands, or viral invasions.

Though humans have around 20,000 genes, with each gene a formula for making a specific protein, gene switches have an even more influential role, activating or suppressing one or more genes at any given instance. The gene-switching molecules are the true decision makers of the cell with the genes simply creating RNA orders going out into the cell. Millions of gene and gene-switching combinations would take place even if the whole system operated randomly or spontaneously. Instead, the millions of gene-switching molecules—also inherited, and which take up 90% of the DNA string—are just as correlated in their logical relationships as the genes themselves, and if destabilized by random mutation, the cell would "crash and burn" without this kind of air traffic controller cohesion. Consider the following report coming out of the University of Washington in 2012:

> *The locations of millions of DNA 'switches' that dictate how, when, and where in the body different genes turn on and off have been identified by a research team led by the University of Washington in Seattle. Genes make up only 2 percent of the human genome and were easy to spot, but the on/off switches controlling those genes were encrypted within the remaining 98 percent of the genome. Without these switches, called regulatory DNA, genes are inert.*

For more on this, read the recent reports coming out of the ENCODE project tasked with researching the human genome.

More so, in the face of the above, even if *spontaneous, synchronized mutations across DNA strands* could even occur in a single cell, they would have to occur over and over again in the exact manner across the entire human population to result in, for instance, a particular breast cancer type called *estrogen sensitive cancer* that 70 percent of breast cancer patients contract. For anyone to intellectually hold onto *universally identical mass mutations happening "spontaneously" among all beings across the vast human species* as the root cause of estrogen sensitive breast cancer constitutes conceptual folly in my opinion.

But that was exactly what the Hartford breast surgeon claimed while we sat in his office: *spontaneous mutation* as the root cause of Laura's condition. And the best schools in America trained him to say so.

This pronouncement stunned me as it left his lips, and I remain stunned.

So, if you dismiss *spontaneous cancer occurrence across one out of every eight woman in America as the root cause of breast cancer,* as I do, then you instead have to envision a specific agent that causes a good, specialized cell—like a lung, prostate, colon, or breast cell—to have its DNA altered right under its very nose.

I'll now offer a more plausible explanation (again, in my opinion).

The Viral Theory of Cancer

Gazillions of viruses exist everywhere, laying siege to every plant and animal on Earth, constantly invading cells, looking for new homes to flourish and multiply in. Organic beings, such as humans, have two lines of defense to fight off these viruses: the cell's immediate response, and the body's "search and destroy" immune system squads.

For example, internally, the cell initiates chemical responses to blunt the virus's attempt to penetrate, blocking the "receptors" on the cell wall membrane that viruses attach themselves to. If a virus is tricky enough to penetrate the cell's membrane, the cell has "personal bodyguard" proteins that identify alien threats with other cell proteins coming in to crush the poor virus just caught. If the cell cannot keep up against the onslaught, a single virus out of thousands may make its way to the center of the cell where it penetrates the nucleus membrane housing the cell's precious DNA and RNA library, or during the copy step as stem cells convert into specialized cells.

Once inside the nucleus, the virus takes over — similar to a bank robber — directing RNA to go out into the cell factory and construct a bunch of SPECIAL "viral" proteins and bring them back into the nucleus. Inside the nucleus, the proteins assemble into thousands of "lifeless" viral drones, á la *Star Wars*, sitting dormant inside of the nucleus chamber. Once the drones are built, duplicated viral DNA strings from the original, perpetrating virus fill the assembled drones to bring them to "life"... err, rather, "activity." And while building a new army of, say, 20,000 viruses (the usual outcome), the perpetrator virus may attempt to infiltrate the cell's DNA making the cell itself cancerous.

Ugly, but it happens some of the time!

Let's consider the HPV virus. Worldwide, HPV is the most common sexually transmitted infection in adults; more than 80 percent of the world's women (3 billion women) will have contracted at least one strain of HPV by age fifty. Most of the 3 billion women infected with HPV will *not* have complications from the HPV virus, as "only" 275,000 people per year die of related HPV *cancer*, around 0.9 % of the infected base. This gives you an idea on the rarity of a virus to get as far as to actually cause cancer. But some do.

The Viral Theory Elaborated

Mechanically, *viral* DNA "strands" are simply infused, wholesale, into the cell's DNA probably during cell division, or during the copy step as stem cells convert into specialized cells. This is similar to replacing one management team with another after a corporate, political, or military takeover. When a DNA infusion transpires, a normal, "assigned" cell ("assigned" to do a job such as performing as a lung cell) is no longer switched to operate according to the rules of cell specialization and programmed death or division (that is, it ignores die commands). It is now a cancer cell.

These cancer cells do not die, and they can suddenly *metastasize*, that is, change forms, such as when breast cancer turns into bone cancer. In addition, cancer cells hate oxygen and love acid, just like viruses. All the behavioral elements of cancer comprise the very traits of viruses.

The ability to metastasize must be rooted in the ability of all cells to copy switch settings during cell division. With *metastasis*, instead of copying one's own settings, the new cell copies another's settings the way stem cells copy the switch settings of the cell they are replacing.

Of course, a well-behaved healthy cell would never copy another cell type's settings during cell division. Only stem cells and cancer cells copy the configuration of others.

Beyond the viral-infected cell itself, which is fighting alone night and day to survive, the body brings its massive immune system to bear to kill off viruses skulking around in the bloodstream and to kill off any unfortunate cell unable to repulse the viral attack; in effect annihilating the badly infected cell and the whole 20,000 strong viral newborns living inside. When cells become this sick to the point where they house 20,000 new viruses waiting to explode onto the scene, the debilitated cell releases last-gasp "SOS." molecules into the bloodstream. These "scented" molecules attract outside immune system cells like T-cells or killer cells to come in and do the dirty work of killing off the infected cell. Let's call it "assisted suicide."

Good riddance!

So if viruses continually bombard the body, then why doesn't everyone have cancer?

The answer: Everyone *does* have cancer, but most bodies, especially younger bodies, possess the strength to keep the viral assault in check.

The body functions as a garden where daily weeding must take place to keep it from, well, "death by weed." In the case of cancer cells, if the body does not destroy errant cells in a timely fashion, they multiply unchallenged and form tumor colonies first in the thousands, then in the millions, then into the billions, and even into the *trillions* of cells. The isolated immune system cells flowing through the blood and lymph systems cannot keep up with the explosion of multiplying cancer cells. The budding tumors initially feed off of the tiny blood and lymph *capillaries* feathered among the healthy cells where they came from, but as the tumors grow, they envelop major blood and lymph *vessels* to co-opt voluminous sources of nutrients, squeezing out the healthy cells. And then it's off to the races!

At some point cancer cannot be stopped. It consumes all of the nutrients of the body until the victim suffers emaciation at the cellular level and finally expires of starvation and oxygen deprivation.

You might find the following study enlightening regarding viruses and their obsession with the DNA within host cells: **Retrovirus Theory on Cancer**

A research report titled, "Roles of Endogenous Retroviruses in Early Life Events," published by *Trends in Microbiology* describes how viral DNA sometimes becomes implanted within the DNA library of sperm and egg cells. While most viral attacks on cells come and go, the researchers believe that over millions of years, some viruses attacking sperm and egg cells manage to permanently plant their DNA inside of these reproduction cells so that the virus's DNA gets passed along as part of the species it successfully invaded. Examination of human DNA points to around 100,000 such cases of viral DNA tucked away within our cells. Though not much is known of the role of foreign DNA in our everyday lives, this research presents compelling evidence that viruses routinely penetrate our DNA libraries and trigger cancers.

Also, before moving on, please consider yet another theory on how cancer starts.

Stem Cell Theory of Cancer

A theory on cancer cites deformed stem cells as a possible cause. Like other cancer theories, damaged DNA is involved, but with the stem cell theory the cancerous DNA is not formed by mature cells during cell division but inside immature stem cells living among the mature cells.

According to the stem cell theory, DNA perversion inside a stem cell causes it to blast out an endless string of "daughter" stem cells that build into tumors. The daughter cells do not multiply; they simply do not die. If this theory holds, it means that each incident of cancer has two different cell types: blaster cells and daughter cells, each possibly needing separate plans to control them. The blaster cells, though, must consume vast amounts of sugar (glucose) to generate this kind of output.

The theory begins with all adult cell types in the body — lung, breast, colon, skin, blood, and so on — having immature "tissue-specific" stem cells living among their mature counterparts. This way, if mature cells are damaged, the nearby tissue-specific stem cells can come out of their dormant state and quickly matriculate into a mature state thereby replacing the damaged cells. Under normal conditions, tissue-specific stem cells remain dormant until needed.

The stem cell cancer theory claims that rather than staying dormant, perverted stem cells go on a wild "blaster" reproduction streak with daughter off-springs causing the buildup of tumors. Even if the tumor is surgically removed, but the rogue, proliferating blaster stem cells are not killed off, the tumor will grow back.

OK, now that we *might* know what we're up against, what's next?

The Cytomegalo Virus

Finally in 2019 further insight into the viral theory surfaced.

In the Acknowledgements section at the beginning of the book, I credited Doctor Blaylock for his deep research into the role of latent (dormant) viruses that cause and drive cancer. In 2019, here is what he reported:

> *Recent studies have found 100 percent incidence of cytomegalovirus in breast cancer tumors, and 94 percent incidence in the lymph nodes draining these cancers.*

This very complex virus encodes more than 750 proteins, many of which play a role in converting normal stem cells into cancer stem cells – thus driving cancer invasion and suppression of anticancer immunity.

The inflammation triggered by these viruses …

Is the primary stimulus for activation of latent cytomegalovirus infections, as once the virus is activated (and reproducing), immune cells dramatically increase the pro-inflammatory enzymes within the tumor's microenvironment.

This inflammation is crucial for sustained tumor cell proliferation.

Natural anti-viral treatments to counter both the virus and the inflammatory response include high-quality Nano Curcumin and Nano Boswellia extracts (Nano means super refined for easy absorption). Doctor Blaylock recommends a product called *Nano Curcumin Plus* which has both compounds. He adds:

Most importantly, unlike chemotherapy and antiviral drugs, a person can take these natural compounds for a lifetime.

The Mayo Clinic opines as follows: *Curcumin is thought to have antioxidant properties, which means it may decrease swelling and inflammation. It's being explored as a cancer treatment in part because inflammation appears to play a role in cancer.*

Part III

More Ups and Downs

Chapter 7

Detoxing with Biological Dentistry

*A*s noted a few chapters ago, the time came for Laura and me to meet the biological dentist. Before this meeting, besides everything I just explained in the preceding chapters, I discovered the following about the field of biological dentistry itself. Fundamentally, biological dentists believe that disturbances in the mouth (the top anchor of the Energy Meridians) and oral bone bacteria are more harmful to your health than mainstream dentistry realizes or understands.

I find it ironic the way mainstream dentistry makes a big deal about gum disease— how microbe toxins in the gum enter the bloodstream and cause conditions such as hardening of the arteries and heart disease. Yet for some reason, mainstream dentistry does not even want to consider that bacteria colonies incubating inside old root canals might secrete other toxins into the bloodstream enabling cancer. Biological dentists on the other hand swear by this last proposition.

They reason as follows: With root canals, the practitioner digs out the main canal and backfills it with a sealant. Before the main canal is destroyed by this procedure and while still alive, it feeds thousands of tiny, microscopic, side fibrous channels that carry nerve, blood, and lymph support to the whole inner tooth (you probably did not know this). By carving out the main channel, the root canal procedure "kills" the tooth outright — right there on the spot — separating all of the side provisioning fibers from the main canal. The strategy supposes that even in a dead state, the tooth's dense bone will remain in the jaw and not decay allowing you to use the tooth as if it were still alive.

Biological dentists cite a few things in response to this line of thinking:

How long do you really expect a dead tooth wedged in your jaw not to create problems? Root canals are a recent phenomenon, and the jury remains out on unforeseen, long-term consequences.

The canal sealant eventually gets old and shrinks enough to form pathways for micro-bacteria to slither into the tooth. They multiply and form colonies inside the abandoned side channels.

Every time you bite down, toxins from these bacterial colonies get squeezed out and swallowed spreading through the body. In turn, saliva is sucked in, bringing needed nutrients back to the bacterial colonies. Whereas toxins from gum disease affect the heart, biological dentists believe that toxins from tooth disease affect soft tissues like breast tissue.

Even if the body can tolerate the toxins (many people fare well with root canals), still, because the Life Energy

Meridians all end up in the mouth, root canals can also impinge energy supplies down the line.

OK, great, I get the theory. I explain the topic to Laura, and off we go on another highway to meet the biological dentist, to hear his ideas in the specific case of Laura's number 3 and number 4 teeth. Perhaps her long-lasting number 3 tooth infection years ago generated the toxins that made her breast tissue vulnerable to viral cancer. The ninety-minute drive to the dentist offers a somber ambiance. So far, our "journey down the yellow brick road" has made us quiet people. But on the drive down, we discuss where we are and project what might come of the upcoming biological dentist meeting.

The biological dentist proves an interesting man. He was a former air force dentist who must have a lot of scientist in him, enough science to try and find out what works on a repeated basis, and if it works, to run with it even if the reasons why it works remain, at least currently, theoretical. Doctor Breiner named his thriving practice Whole Body Dentistry. At one point, the American Dental Association (ADA) spent seven years trying to shut him down because of his views on mercury fillings, root canals, and so on, all of which counter ADA policies.

We stayed there for hours. After presenting our current situation and our self-healing plan framework, he started by taking a sample of Laura's plaque, which we all examined under a microscope and observed the world of bacteria alive in her mouth. He specifically drew the sample to hunt for specific "bad" bacteria types stemming from tooth and bone infections. He next took a panoramic x-ray of Laura's entire jaw to see where issues from the past might still remain. They appeared evident only in teeth number 3 and number 4, just as we told him. He recommended removing the number 4 tooth that had been treated with a root canal a year ago. We expected this and agreed to do it; later, however, we changed our minds.

VOLL Testing

Then the interesting stuff started, the testing for toxins in the body: heavy metals, pesticides, chemical pollutants, bacterial by-products and fungi. He used a VOLL system, something I had researched that had been universally and severely ridiculed by all commentators, yet never explained.

Here is the theory behind the VOLL device. The VOLL machine, a custom computer apparatus, includes a brass pointer wired from the computer's sending side and a brass pipe wired to the returning side. The machine sends low voltage electricity through your body to measure resistance caused by chemicals buried in the body (you cannot feel the electrical current). The procedure pokes the pointer into one hand while you hold the returning pipe in the other hand creating a circuit, starting with the computer, flowing through your body and returning back to the computer. In other words, a "clean" electric current (at a very low voltage) delivered by the pointer rod easily makes its way through your body to connect up with the receiving pipe held by your other hand.

Next, now that a clean circuit passes through your body with minor, yet measured, resistance, the clean current is infused with "electronic spectrum" imprints of various carcinogens. *Spectrum* means the electrical manifestation of a discrete object such as mercury or fluoride. Elements and other objects have specific electrical spectrums. Sounds, for example, have spectrum shapes we store on compact discs as "music." Every discrete object out there possesses a unique electrical spectrum, the way every snowflake is unique.

When we add one of these toxic spectrum images into the clean current passing through the body, the augmented current slows down because of the resistance provided by actual toxic matter in the body pulling the electronic spectrum toward it. If, for example, we add the electronic spectrum for mercury to the electrical current entering the body, and real mercury already exists in the body perhaps derived from your mercury fillings and the consumption of certain fish over your lifetime, then the electrical current slows down based upon the degree of real mercury it encounters. A high level of contaminant mercury in the body will virtually stop the current in its tracks. The VOLL machine shows the decay in current, which signals the magnitude of the toxin in the body.

A Five-Step and Five-Month Detox Program

The outcome of this benchmarking step became a five-month program to rid Laura's body of deeply imbedded toxins, one class of toxins at a time. Month 1 would target respiratory pollutants, month 2 ingested heavy metals, and so forth. To achieve these monthlong cleansings, the doctor imprinted electronic spectrums of the toxins into a vial of water—similar to imprinting a CD—instructing Laura to take a capful of this augmented water each day. He did not put real mercury into the water, just the electronic spectrum of mercury.

To get a grip on this, think of this analogy: While Earth's gravity pulls on the moon, the moon, too possesses gravity and pulls on Earth at a *reduced level*, but *pull* it does. Likewise, the mercury image inside the water, tiny though it may be, nevertheless pulls on the *real* mercury embedded in the body, and the *image* of the energy DRAWS THE PHYSICAL MERCURY OUT!

Hmm…we will have to digest this claim.

Upon concluding the biological dentistry episode, Laura and I drive home emotionally shattered. Just *what* had we conjured? On the way home, we stop en route in Waterbury, Connecticut for dinner at Diorio, a wonderful Italian restaurant I frequented over the years. I remember that we ordered sautéed broccoli rabe and Caesar salads, that we sat, quietly, and that finally we conversed trying to assimilate what we had just heard from the Brave New World of Homeopathic Medicine.

Homeopathic medicine simply means using the same, or "homeo," substance as medicine that one is going after as the cause of the suffering, or "pathic." *Like cures like*. Many incorrectly apply this phrase to all naturalistic and organic cures.

One other thing; the biological dentist gave us the phone number of Dr. Robert Bard, a diagnostic doctor in New York City, who could take a three-dimensional picture of Laura's tumors using a special sonogram system. This would allow us to follow the growth or the retreat of the tumors in great detail.

Dental Hygiene

Doctor Breiner had made a deep impression about the degree of exposure the body has to viruses and bacteria residing in the teeth, jaws, and gums. As mentioned, we had examined samples taken from Laura's mouth under his microscope so that he could gauge the intensity of microbe activity and look for specific bacteria that do not belong in the mouth.

At home, we ramped up our dental hygiene program to a three-step process: 1) *electric toothbrush* to clean exterior areas, followed by 2) *flossing* to break up microbe colonies between the teeth and below the gum line, followed by 3) *water pick cleanse* to flush everything out sending it all down the drain.

This proved a no-brainer. Removing billions of microbes from your mouth on a daily basis enables the immune system to focus on other body zones.

Toxicity and Water

Another thing that really sank in after meeting the biological dentist: Addressing toxicity in the body begins with an understanding of *water*.

Considering that cells are comprised mainly of water, that same water probably constitutes more than 70 percent of the human body. Every toxic element inside your water supply finds its way to each of the trillions of cells in your body. The water you drinks proves critical toward keeping the body's cells contamination-free. When we got home from the visit, after looking toxins in the eye vis-à-vis the dentist's VOLL machine, we immediately switched to bottled water that boasted a clean lab report.

Mercury and Fluoride

I also read Doctor Briener's book, *Whole Body Dentistry*, which revealed other key facts such as the following:

Over decades, we inhale mercury molecules millions of times from the mercury vapors escaping from our dental fillings, and we ingest fluoride, another toxin that we foolishly drink with our water.

These toxins, after years of consumption, stay buried deep inside of us. The crazy thing? Both mercury and fluoride are poisons, yet we go out of our way to ingest them on a perpetual basis.

With mercury, besides dental fillings, carnivorous fish—such as swordfish—contain large quantities of it. Every species of fish ingests some mercury as over time modern society continues to discharge significant levels of mercury into the water supply. Ground-feeder breeds such as sole and flounder ingest the least amounts of mercury.

Medium-sized fish eating these smaller fish ingest the ground feeder's mercury, accumulating higher levels.

Larger fish that eat the medium fish collect even more mercury concentrations, and so on. At the top of the food chain, swordfish, for instance, contain forty times the amount of mercury as do the ground feeders.

Moving on to fluoride, we mix it in with our drinking water to fight bacteria in our mouths, which means that it reaches every cell in our body—just to find our teeth. This crazy practice started after World War II and later stopped all over the world—*except in America!* And these constitute only two of the many carcinogens we remain exposed to. The biological dentist has electronic spectrums for *500* known toxins.

Immune System Empowerment

Toxicity exists *everywhere*, but there *is* good news. If you have lived forty or sixty years, your body has forty to sixty years of absorbed toxicity hidden away, BUT you can more or less return to Square One — the way your body arrived at birth — through comprehensive detox efforts.

According to the Centers for Disease Control (The CDC), 210 million Americans out of an overall national population of 313 million still ingest fluoridated water daily.

Laura did the fourteen-day enzyme-led detox to get things started, and then did five, one-month-each homeopathic, energy-led regimens to remove the deep stuff. Toxins cause free radicals and are acidic, squeezing oxygen out of the bloodstream. Toxins next divert the immune system to chase after them rather than staying focused on the disease at hand, causing a chronic inflammation response. Once detoxification begins, you can take additional steps to further boost the body's oxygen levels, its energy levels, and the overall vigor of the immune system (described in "Part V — Boosting the Body").

Chapter 8

News...and Bad News

*B*ack home, we receive a call saying that Laura's nutrition report has arrived. We go down to see our naturopath doctor to learn the results.

The Nutrition Report

For each mineral or vitamin, the lab report shows where your mineral or vitamin level sits in comparison to the general population. If, say, your B12 level as achieved through daily digestion and absorption resides in the bottom 10 percent of humanity, then you need to start taking B12 supplements. The report tells you the dosage you need to get you to an adequate level.

Laura ranked low in five areas, so she began taking supplements at home adding these into her daily intake program. The regimen dictated that she take some supplements at specific times of the day or before or after a meal. Laura designed a "when and how much" chart that scheduled both the supplements and the homeopathic waters. It would soon expand to coordinate the immune-system bolstering and cancer-infiltration elements of our budding self-healing plan.

Iodine

A funny thing about the nutrient report; it did *not* include an assessment of iodine. Iodine deficiency correlates highly to occurrences of breast cancer. Because of this recognized correlation, iodine must play a role in the healthy operation of the unique female cells (breast and ovary cells) designed to divide during menstrual cycles.

As national author Doctor David Brownstein describes: "The breasts contain the third-highest iodine concentration in the body after the thyroid gland and the ovaries. Iodine deficiency in the breast can manifest as fibrocystic breast disease and breast cancer." I recommend Dr. David Brownstein's, book, *"Iodine: Why You Need It, Why You Can't Live Without It."*

I researched suppliers and purchased an iodine supplement.

The kineologist handling Laura's energy health did more research and set a moderate dose (Japanese diets have even higher levels – seaweed). Iodine is an *essential* (must be ingested) ingredient for female sex cells, and I attribute this corrected deficiency as one of the contributors to Laura's success. However, I'm not certain about the following, but I did find it compelling: Iodine—applied to wounds—kills viruses. Because a lack of iodine correlates to an increased occurrence of breast cancer, maybe the breast cells ward off viral bugs using iodine. While researching breast cancer topics, I ran into a corollary finding on male prostate chemistry that you might find interesting.

Just as female tissue employs iodine (a poison) to regulate organ health, prostate tissue employs zinc (a poison)—fifteen times as much zinc as found elsewhere in the body—to fend off viral and cancerous development within that gland.

The body is tricky, using poisons in a controlled manner to do its bidding.

First, the *Good* News: 3-D Sonograms

Our date for the 3-D sonogram trip to New York City came up (not to be confused with the other New York City trip to see the Columbia laser doctor scheduled a week later). Dr. Bard, the 3-D sonogram pioneer and breast and prostate cancer specialist, administered the sonogram in the normal manner, the difference being that this specialized sonogram dispersed 120 discrete sonogram waves into different depths of the breast and wrote each deeper image to disk. Back in the doctor's office, a software package written by General Electric assembled the different depth images and compiled a 3-D image of the tumor, and the 3-D image could be spun around to examine each side of the tumor.

Two things came of this:

1) We now had precise measurements of both tumors; their lengths, widths, and depths, to serve as our baseline, and

2) The doctor commented that no big blood vessels entered either tumor so that the tumors would not have the nutrients to become aggressive in the short

term. He did point out that the large tumor was approaching a vessel, and if it could grow around the vessel, then it would co-opt it, launching an aggressive growth phase.

We left feeling confident that we could go all-out with the diet and cleansing approach along with all the other measures I had come up with and put off standard surgery for now (though we still held interest in the laser idea). We made an appointment to have the tumors measured again ten weeks hence.

And Now, the Big Letdown...

I have not really brought this up until now, but stress, fatigue, and worry do not well serve people trying to arrest cancer. When in distress, your body's nervous system puts everything on high alert. You assume the classic "fight or flight" stance. At this point, your body's immune and repair systems effectively become shuttered until the body broadcasts certain "all clear" hormones throughout the bloodstream directing cells to finally "rest and recover." (I will discuss the fight or flight response versus rest and recovery topic further in the "Boosting Energy" chapter.)

I only bring up the role of stress now to put the following event in context: The Columbia Presbyterian Laser Therapy option (mentioned earlier) proved a washout with heavy fallout on Laura's psyche. As I mentioned, I spoke to the Columbia doctor's office multiple times, attained an appointment date, and had all MRIs, regular sonograms, 3-D sonograms, and mammograms sent to the doctor's office as well as the pathology slides (the actual cancer cell samples from the original biopsy) held at Hartford Hospital. Laura and I discussed many times that we should not get our hopes up as the "Laser Zapper" treatment (as we called it) remained experimental, and we might not even be chosen to undergo the treatment. Still, we had mailed in all our stuff, plus I had contacted their office one day earlier to ensure that they had everything they wanted from us.

And then the big day arrives, and we drive almost three hours into Manhattan to get the lowdown. We leave early and stop for salad along the way and again promise each other not to raise our hopes up too high. We realize that if things do not work out, then "it's a long ride home."

We arrive. We park. We find the office. They appear embarrassed to see us saying they tried calling (while we were driving) to tell us we did not qualify. Besides Laura's nine-millimeter tumor, she also had a smaller, four-millimeter tumor, and the funded research program only considered single-tumor cases.

I stayed calm, but knew Laura was beginning to crumble. And that's when it all became surrealistic. They next told us that even if Laura had qualified with a single tumor, their research program still required — get this — 1) a standard lumpectomy to examine the dead tumor zapped by the laser, and 2) a full six weeks of radiation, just in case.

"Who would sign up for this?" I asked, and they replied that so far, twenty-three women *had*. The volunteers gained no advantage personally; they did it to help the program. Apparently research funding for the program came with the lumpectomy and radiation strings attached until a FDA-type of government authority sanctioned the procedure. The procedure, itself, they told us, showed results. Their process destroyed twenty-three tumors without collateral damage to the breast. Ironically, the collateral damage only came later with the lumpectomy and radiation that the program demanded to protect its own agenda. They apologized, again for not making all of this clear during the previous and various phone calls and asked if we wanted to sign up for a regular lumpectomy.

Our reply?

"No thanks."

Back in the elevator, back in the parking lot, paying for the parking, driving past the George Washington Bridge... and Laura continues to slowly crumble....We keep talking to deflate her anger and stress, but it remains a three-hour ride home. Now, at least, it became official. We would stand on our own. NO MEDICAL INTERVENTION CRUTCHES! This resolution, though, meant digging deeper into the body's biology and charting our own strategies...without regret.

A "Regular" Dental Visit

But first, one more topic requires attention before we solidify our cancer plan direction: the idea of extracting Laura's number 4 tooth that had an undergone a root canal. Laura was complaining about pain coming from the bridge attached to teeth number 4 and number 2 (number 3, if you remember, had been pulled eight years ago). We assume the pain is coming from the number 4 tooth, which underwent a root canal one year ago.

But we were wrong.

Our regular dentist poked around and determined the pain came from tooth number 2, a supposedly *good* tooth. He took an x-ray of tooth number 2 that revealed no evidence of any issues whatsoever, though the tooth still hurt. We drilled the bridge down to reduce contact pressure and left it at that, though months later Laura still felt moderate pain coming from tooth number 2. Considering all the moving parts to Laura's health puzzle, we decided to do nothing with the teeth for now. Instead, we would concentrate on shrinking the tumors. If the teeth pulled almost a decade ago proved part of the root cause of the cancer, then we would decide upon this at a later time after we successfully arrested the cancer. We canceled the number 4 tooth extraction procedure agreed upon back in the biological dentist's office and ignored the number 2 tooth pain...for now.

Ok, now let's shrink some tumors.

Part IV

Diet and Digestion

Chapter 9

How Diet Enables Cancer

*A*s said in the book's introduction, three principle rails traverse the self-healing path: (1) *diet* (deprive the cancer of sugar while nourishing all of the body's good cells); (2) *tumor infiltration* (poison the tumors); and (3) *immune system empowerment* (free the immune system from toxins and then boost its energy level). Here in chapter 9, we conceptually explore how diet works with an outline of the specific diet explained later in chapter 10. Chapter 9 is a long chapter, but filled it with important physiological and biological elements including frameworks on digestion, stimulants, fats, nutrients, sugars, toxins, and more.

Let's begin with a look at digestion starting with the food we eat and excrete through the digestive tract and followed by a synopsis of how the body processes food once it's inside the bloodstream—and what can happen when this system becomes either flawed or overextended.

Digestion in a Nutshell

Because our biochemical cell factories interact with molecules and not directly, say, with carrots or chicken nuggets, our bodies must break down the things we eat to the molecular level to provide value in the world of cells. A carrot gets broken down in stages starting with your teeth and saliva. Then stomach acids, duodenum bile, and pancreas enzymes bombard it, all before it enters a twenty-two-foot-long small intestine where "good" microbes break things down further.

Inside of our intestines, trillions of good bacteria reside ingesting all the food sent their way. Once ingested, the bacteria's "body" churns the incoming food and excretes it. The excreted molecules are more refined than the source molecules allowing them to be absorbed through the intestine walls into the bloodstream. Also, the bacteria excrete special molecules, like vitamin B12, that our bodies need.

It is hard to accept, but there are many times as many digestive bacteria in our intestines then there are cells in our entire body!

Once the nutrients are reduced through this elaborate chemical and bacterial assembly line, they finally enter the bloodstream through the small intestine walls, and anything that is not absorbed passes on through a valve to the large intestine for eventual excretion. Great!

Absorbed nutrients next flow directly to the liver, which converts the nutrients into even finer molecules that the cells can absorb before they are transported by a vein to the heart. From the heart, the nutrient-laden blood passes through the lungs to fetch oxygen and is sent back to the heart again via a different valve, and from there the heart pushes both nutrients and oxygen to the body's cells. Yikes! That's a lot of trouble to go through for a carrot or a chicken nugget! Who made this wacky system up?

To provide perspective on the effort the body exerts to break down ingested food, consider this: Generally, most people ingest two-to-four quarts of food and drink per day, yet the body injects an additional eight quarts of "digestive fluids" into the digestive tract to move things along and break the food down. In addition, we swallow one to two quarts of saliva per day; stomach acids contribute another two to three quarts; the duodenum receives two quarts of bile created by the liver and pancreatic enzymes daily; and the small intestine weighs in with two more quarts of "lubricant" fluid.

The blood and lymph vessels entwined around the small and large intestines reabsorb almost all of the ten to fourteen quarts of fluid—both ingested and bodily supplied—leaving only a subset of fluid actually excreted (sweat and kidney filtration actually maintain fluid equilibrium inside the body).

The digestive fluid basically comprises a closed-end system orchestrated by a strong liver that is able to scrub all of the incoming digestive fluids and recycle them.

Stimulants Bypass Digestion

Cocaine, for one, doesn't need to pass through these hoops. Once snorted, it passes through nasal membranes inside the nose and enters the bloodstream directly rushing instantaneously to the brain. White sugar, caffeine, and alcohol also bypass the standard hoops. Similar to cocaine, we foist these upon the body without digestion's filtering channels. Once swallowed, they arrive already in the "broken-down," micro-molecule form, and the bloodstream quickly absorbs them whether or not the body even wants more sugar, caffeine, or alcohol.

Direct access to the bloodstream remains the trait of all (let's call them) "power bar" substances. Unwanted power bars, similar to other unwanted "visitors," do not simply proceed to the large intestine. Once these power bar substances enter the bloodstream, internal organs and every single cell undertake the job of purging these unwanted substances from the body. Instead, now that the "power bar" molecules reside within, they grow into a big, complex deal, creating a rippling effect throughout the system.

However, something like brown rice is quite the opposite. Inside the rice's inner kernel resides a bit of carbohydrate, minerals, and vitamins that the body actually wants, but seven fibrous sheaths enclose the inner kernel. The body works hard to dig through the seven layers and in the process of digging, ONLY THE MOLECULES WANTED BY THE BODY ARE ISOLATED FOR ABSORBTION, including the rice's *soluble* fiber, its minerals, vitamins, and some of its inner kernel energy. Actually, the body does not want most of the rice—including its nonsoluble fiber—yet even this plays a role by binding with other unwanted food and by scraping against the intestine walls similar to a sanitation truck clearing your "street."

Now, take white rice. All seven layers of fiber were stripped bare, leaving a bleached, inner kernel stripped of many key mineral and vitamin molecules that are now almost pure carbohydrate molecules for the body to encounter.

Once inside, the body quickly breaks down carbohydrates into sugar molecules, which get absorbed unconditionally, similar to those of a power bar. All that remains? Unwanted sugar, but no vitamins or minerals; only clogged intestines.

This situation itself does not cause cancer, but on a chronic basis, surely it sets the table, nicely.

Let's go into more detail. This way you can converse with doctors, nutritionists, and the other experts you will encounter on your journey.

The Blood and Lymph Circulatory Systems

We possess two circulatory systems: the blood and lymphatic systems, with parallel blood and lymph vessels running throughout the body. Whereas the heart pumps blood through a close-ended *circulatory* system, the lymph passively "oozes" from each cell into open, *one-way* lymphatic pathways. Simple movements of the body then nudge lymph plasma along through lymph vessels. The slow-moving lymph trickles into the bloodstream through yet another valve near the heart.

Note: The lymph system, which clears debris from the body, requires exercise to move things along. Laura's six days per week of formal exercise via the karate program was a key to her success. Massage helps as well.

Why *two* systems?

Basically, blood delivers nutrients and oxygen to the cells in a real-time, no-delay manner, whereas lymph performs auxiliary functions at a slower pace allowing the blood system to remain focused on the moment-by-moment delivery of essential fuels. The lymph system performs specialty jobs such as collecting waste from cells, delivering white immune cells to desired locations, and transporting fat (packaged as *triglycerides)* from the intestines to the bloodstream.

Tissue Fluid and Osmosis

Every one of the body's 100 trillion cells has access to both blood and lymph services. These capillaries do not touch the cells themselves but remain in contact with "tissue fluid" that surrounds each cell. Through *osmosis*, cells import and export substances from the fluid chamber, and the blood and lymph membranes do the same dance via osmosis to keep the tissue fluid chamber neutral.

Osmosis — The ability of a fluid or materials to pass through a *semipermeable membrane* thus equalizing the concentrations of materials on either side of the membrane.

An important note: *In this osmosis-led mechanism, the cells have no choice in what they absorb.* For example, if alcohol exists in the bloodstream, the blood capillary membrane will push the alcohol into the cell's tissue fluid chamber for the cell to absorb to create equal concentrations of alcohol inside and outside of the cell wall. The cell exports alcohol only when the tissue fluid chamber no longer contains alcohol, that is, after you drink a lot of water and clear the alcohol from your system. The same goes for *all* toxins. If they exist in the tissue chamber, the cell will take them in to create parity of the substance inside and outside of the cell membrane wall.

Abusing the System

With the above in mind, consider the multi-cup coffee drinker where caffeine flows to all 100 trillion cells. As the kidneys clear the caffeine from the bloodstream, all 100 trillion cells start to push their caffeine back out to the tissue fluid and from there to the capillaries. Then the drinker ingests the next cup of coffee and the process repeats itself. After three to four cups, the body spends the day pumping caffeine in and out of all of these cells, exhausting the system.

Now that we know what *not* to do—consume caffeine, alcohol, sugar, and drugs— let's visualize the *original* design for the body's performance.

Stimulants are big "no-no's" with cancer-fighting diets. Health-wise, cells have much more important things to do— such as killing viruses—than to pump useless chemicals in and out of themselves all day long.

Separate Digestion Steps for Fats, Oils and all Other Nutrients

As already described, digestion of incoming food involves a two-step process: (1) *mechanical* alteration, or the raw ingestion and breakdown of food by the mouth, stomach, and duodenum, and (2) *chemical* alteration of ingested materials by the intestines and liver to create molecules actually usable by cells. A lot happens to ready nutrient molecules to attach and then pass through the body's 100 trillion cells.

Whether the food presents a fat or oil (meat) or other (a carrot), the digestion process starts out the same way.

Chewing and saliva begin the process.

Next, the stomach muscles churn the food, mixing in acids, which convert the raw food into a semiliquid substance called "chime."

Chime then enters the duodenum, where the gallbladder injects bile (the liver actually creates bile and stores it in the gallbladder until it is needed to digest a meal). *Bile*, an antiseptic, is interesting first in that it kills the microbes that arrive with the food, and second, bile is super-alkaline, neutralizing the temporary acidity of the chime (remember, the body does not want acid).

The pancreas then supplies the duodenum with digestive enzymes designed to separate fat clumps in the chime and provide insulin for glucose distribution. Fat raises a special challenge to the body. Fat tends to clump together and cannot mix with water, and water is our centerpiece constituting 70 percent of our bodies.

To solve this fat/water conflict, pancreas enzymes injected into the duodenum latch onto the animal fat molecules to keep them from sticking to each other.

The ability of one animal (mankind) to live off the bodies of outside animals and plants can be boiled down to this: The digestive track reduces the incoming fat and protein molecules structured for the outside organism into smaller building block molecules that human cells reassemble to suit their own purposes. Animal proteins are broken down into a slew of amino acids, which human cells draw upon to form human protein structures ordered up by human DNA and RNA templates.

Upon leaving the duodenum, the chemically separated fat molecules, proteins, and vitamin nutrients enter the twenty-two-foot-long small intestines where what we call "good bacteria" break them down further.

This relationship between the bacteria in our "gut" and the nutrients we need emphasizes why we must take care not to decimate the good bacteria with harmful drugs, including chemotherapy. Conversely, we often see probiotics prescribed to nurture the good bacteria.

Strings of blood and lymph capillaries surround the twenty-two-foot-long intestine cell walls waiting to absorb the incoming molecular nutrients predigested by the good bacteria.

The fat components, however, remain too big to fit through the red blood capillary membranes, so the more porous lymph capillaries pick up the fat droplets. All the other smaller nutrients enter the red blood capillaries and next go straight to the liver for further processing. Fat goes the other way, through the lymph system.

Let's follow what happens to fat.

Processing Fat

Upon entering the lymph system, the separated fat droplets reconfigure to create human *triglycerides* — fat packets. For example, upon eating some tuna, the incoming fish triglycerides from the tuna first broken down into tiny fat droplets are reconfigured by intestinal cells for the triglyceride design of the human body.

Fat, in triglyceride form, stands ready to be metabolized into keytone (not glucose) energy packets by the liver to feed the body. The triglyceride packets drift through the lymph vessels and get dumped into the bloodstream (at that lymph/blood gateway near the heart). The bloodstream, in turn, exposes the triglyceride packets to the body's fat cells. The fat cells unconditionally absorb the excess triglycerides storing them away until told to release them when you're very hungry. We have a fixed set of fat cells in our bodies;

they simply expand, as necessary, to deal with overloads of triglycerides inundating the body. Around 10 percent of fat cells die each year but are replaced with a new 10 percent.

Because the fat cell count remains fixed, when you remove fat via liposuction, the fat cells in the treated area disappear for good. However, if you continue to overload the system, other fat cells take up the slack in a "robbing Peter to pay Paul" manner. Your back, rather than your stomach, becomes fat!

Besides warehousing triglycerides, the fat cells operate as a general storage facility for all kinds of excesses floating around the body, such as toxins. This combination of fat and toxins sitting inside of fat cells is why when you start a cancer-effective cleansing diet, you need to follow the diet for as long as it takes (typically two to three months) to "squeeze the stuffing" out of the fat cells, thus eliminating the hidden reserves of fat energy and acidic toxins that are available to the cancer cells.

The Interplay of Sugar and Triglycerides

A related point: When you consume sugar, even fruit sugar, the excess calories from the sugar mean that the body does not yet call out the triglyceride reserves leaving these fat and toxicity reserves intact, thus delaying the effects of the deprivation plan. A website called ReduceTriglycerides. com offers some lucid observations on triglycerides, sugar, and cancer, as follows:

"If you strictly follow a sugar-free diet, a significant drop in your blood triglyceride level should occur in four to six weeks. Unfortunately, many people actually suffer an addiction to sugar, and this includes grains that are rapidly broken down into sugar by the body. Only if you completely avoid all sugar and grains will you eliminate this physical addiction. But for several weeks during the transition, you MUST eat *every* two hours to avoid the symptoms of hypoglycemia."

Remember, cancer cells cannot multiply rapidly without sugar and that the cells that divide the fastest have the highest energy requirements. Yet I am flabbergasted that this simple knowledge — *sugar feeds cancer* — does not prevail as Rule Number One in *any* cancer fight: STOP *eating sugar immediately*."

More Bad News about Sugar

OK, that sends another strong message about sugar, but sugar excess raises another issue: *glycation*.

Glycation: a biochemical process that comes on strong with age, combines sugar with collagen resulting in an inert new molecule. As a result, pure collagen's "antiaging" proteins become depleted throughout the body (in other words, *sugar ages you*).

A web of stringy things made out of a molecule called *collagen* holds our bodies together. We are all Spider Man! But you want elastic collagen rather than stiff collagen fibers running throughout your body. Your skin wrinkles because the proteins needed to produce skin collagen grow scarce because they're busy bonding with excess sugars.

The same thing happens throughout the body. As the antiaging collagen supply dwindles, muscles become less supple; your arteries grow brittle; and so forth. You cannot control the aging process, but you *can* eliminate simple sugars thereby preventing this vitality-producing protein from being neutralized.

OK, all of the above information primarily concerned fat: its special digestion path, how the body uses and stores it, and why sugars prevent the total depletion of fat. More on sugar, collagen, scar tissue, and breast density later in the book.

A note on sugars and PET scans: With PET scans, radioactive sugar is injected intravenously to circulate throughout the whole body. Generally speaking, there are three types of cells that devour sugar—brain, heart, and cancer cells. These then glow on the PET scan monitor because of the radioactive element mixed in with the sugar. Hence, cancer concentrations can be found with tumors of .8 cm or larger. This gives you a feel for the sugar appetite of cancer cells.

The Liver

Now, we must visualize what happens to all other nonfat nutrients entering the bloodstream directly from the intestines. After your intestines, the biggest single organ you have is your liver. It starts on your right side and runs all the way to your stomach on the left connecting back to the digestive tract via its helper organ, the gallbladder (which the liver provides with cholesterol-based bile used to help with digestion).

Why is the liver so big?

It does a lot of work, that's why. I read that it performs five hundred different functions. It mainly scours incoming blood from the intestines looking for newly ingested food, enzymes, glucose, minerals, vitamins, plus circulating triglycerides. Its main functions include the following:

The liver uses the various "B" family of vitamins to refine these raw entities into "bite-sized" nutrient packages that can attach to cell walls.

If the body is not "hungry," the liver stores up the refined nutrients and then slowly drips them into the bloodstream over the next few hours to keep all 100 trillion cells happy.

The liver also manufactures cholesterol. The body uses *cholesterol*, a building-material molecule, to build cell membranes.

Because we have 100 trillion cell membranes, we need a lot of cholesterol. Besides being the "brick and mortar" of cell membrane walls, the body uses cholesterol to create nerve coatings and to formulate steroid hormones that direct the body's organs. Finally, cholesterol helps create bile, which is injected into the duodenum for digestive purposes.

It's everywhere!

HDL cholesterol, the good cholesterol produced by the liver, possesses a great deal of protein. *LDL cholesterol* (the bad cholesterol) mainly possesses fat. *Triglycerides*, mentioned earlier, initially packaged by the lymph system, exist mainly as pure fat packets and are readily converted to ketones.

A big payoff from the self-healing plan diet is that it eliminates excess fat throughout both facets of the digestive system — blood and lymph. Hence, both LDL cholesterol (mainly fat) and triglycerides (pure fat) levels will decline in due course. Laura's triglycerides dropped from 120 to 43.

Everyone always mentions triglycerides when discussing cholesterol, and I am not sure why people officially" bundle them together other than the fat connection. The body forms and uses triglycerides and cholesterol separately inside the body.

Last, the liver serves as a big filter attempting to identify and remove unwanted toxins from the bloodstream. It mixes filtered material with cholesterol to make bile, and pushes this material into the bile sac for storage. When the liver injects bile into the duodenum for digestive purposes, the toxins go with it and work their way down the intestines for excretion.

Poor Diets + Toxins = It All Adds Up

The overall point?

If you abuse your digestive process by flooding your body with stuff it does not want—coffee, fats, refined carbohydrates, raw sugars—then you will constantly work your insides overtime. The likely scenario? You probably (and unwittingly) subject your organs and your universe of cells to the compromise and challenge of dealing with excesses, thus enhancing their exposure to becoming more vulnerable to ever-lurking viruses.

OK, not so good, so let's add toxins into the mix to make things even *worse*.

If food excess itself presents a problem, then consider food excess *plus* toxins. Experts estimate that today thousands of synthetically manufactured chemicals and prescription drugs confront our bodies, chemicals that humans never encountered prior to 1900. For the most part, toxins are acidic, causing free radicals and lower oxygen levels in the body. What mechanism deals with these ugly, oxygen-robbing poisons residing inside your body?

Well, certainly your liver and kidneys get involved as they serve as the main filtering and excretion organs dealing with toxins and nutritional waste. But toxins affect all the other cells, too. Just as the body parks excess triglycerides inside fat cells, it also begins to park all of the toxins inside other cells — say, inside breast cells, for example.

The osmosis dynamic comes into play everywhere between the cells and the blood and lymph streams exchanging both natural and man-made chemicals. Just as the roots of plants mindlessly absorb molecules from the outside world, our cells have no choice but to absorb what surrounds them. And just as alcohol makes you woozy when you absorb it, toxic substances make each cell woozy.

Toxic chemicals compromise the cell's fragile biochemical DNA/RNA communication network by inserting multiple, meaningless chemical signals into the mix. The cell can no longer "think clearly" about how to defend itself against the outside viruses continually pressing against its walls. And so, with defenses down, the viruses gain entry to the cell where they do their worst.

Toxic chemical signals also slow down the immune system cells. In its groggy, oxygen-depleted state, the body nevertheless calls upon immune cells to kill more and more virally infected cells. But alas, the feeble immune cells fall behind, and infected cells remain in play and viruses become emboldened. In some cases, viral assaults go so far as breaching a cell's DNA library and replacing part of the cell's DNA with viral DNA, giving birth to cancer, with an immune system too "fatigued" to do much about it.

The story then continues with colonies of multiplying cancer cells, visible tumors, metastasizing cells...and the eventual death of the host.

Chapter 10

The Self-Healing Diet

Given everything discussed, I tell people that diet stands strong as the centerpiece to the self-healing plan, but other elements such as energy and immune system boosting also play an important role. Twenty-eight years ago with my first wife, diet (in her case, the Japanese diet) existed as the sole element of the plan, and this, by itself, brought her back to life. But understanding has evolved. Diet might provide the battering ram, but the other elements deliver the necessary "knockout force" to ensure its impact. And even more so, the surrounding plan elements help cure you quickly, and further, the full plan helps to relaunch you at a top-of-the-line health and beauty level.

Speaking of beauty, once on the diet, Laura began dropping weight, which caused her concern. Would the weight loss keep going until she shriveled down to nothing? Well, at the five-month mark, she leveled out at 113 pounds, the same weight she carried on our wedding day at twenty-eight years of age. Laura's good friend Audrey, another black belt karate enthusiast, maintains the diet at all times, and she does not have cancer. She just "gets it," and she, too enjoys "perfect" condition with "perfect" looks.

Audrey, by the way, helped Laura get started with the diet showing her where to shop, how to work the juicer, sending us articles, dropping off farm produce, and just providing a steady intellectual and psychological force always moving things forward. As the saying goes: "That's what friends are for."

The diet comprises three principal considerations:

1. Starve the cancer primarily by digesting vegetables thus keeping sugar, carbohydrate, and fat levels as low as possible.
2. Eat foods that produce more alkaline, less acidic digestive responses (for example, kale and sweet potatoes), as alkaline promotes oxygen, which bolsters normal cells and weakens cancer cells.
3. Make certain your limited food diversity nevertheless keeps you nourished, factoring in the need for vitamins, electrolytes, amino acids, omega 3s, and antioxidants.

Actually, the diet appears fairly complicated, especially at first when you must both research and memorize all of the "food rules." If I wrote this book as a strict diet guide, the diet specifics would grow very detailed very quickly.

This chapter instead covers the basics so you can quickly gain orientation and take the first meaningful anticancer steps ASAP in a week's time. After taking the basic steps—the steps that deliver 80 percent of the devastating diet effects against the cancer cells—you can read the big, three-hundred-page cancer diet tomes to really get into the fray.

Use incremental information nuggets described in these in-depth books to fine-tune your diet during months 2, 3, and 4.

Because you will fret as to whether any of this works, you will want to have a few images taken of your tumors along the way to follow the plan's progress.

Laura had her baseline sonogram taken in week 3 of the diagnosis with the first checkpoint 90 days out where they found her larger tumor half of its original size. At the second checkpoint 120 days later, they couldn't find the small tumor at all, and the large tumor had reduced by half once more. These kinds of results can really keep you motivated.

A Good Diet vs. a "Cancer Diet"

The first thing to understand regarding diet: the difference between a good, *balanced diet* that you might follow if you were healthy and a *self- healing diet* where you go the extra lengths necessary to force advancing cancer back into its hole.

For example, many balanced diets include a portion of fruit, yet fruit contains plenty of sugar, so why include it when you're trying to deny cancer cells the multiples of sugar they *crave*? Though fruit offers antioxidants, you can take supplements instead.

Likewise, with acid: acidic substances weakens the body's cells including immune system cells, depriving them of oxygen. Conversely, cancer cells hate alkaline, as alkaline introduces more oxygen. And so enjoying steak (acidic) must wait until you tame the cancer, and kale (alkaline) must become a dietary staple. Because you cross off many things you currently ingest and enjoy from your diet, the diet thus poses a daunting challenge especially early on

---

when through habit, comfort, and even addiction, you will crave the foods you must eliminate. Only time, at least one month of following the diet, can soften this. And at all times, remember the "sugar and acid" rules: *Cancer needs many times the sugar as do normal cells, and acid suppresses oxygen.*

Acidic Causing Substances

A few chapters back, I explained why lemon juice, though acidic, causes an overall alkaline effect on the bloodstream. Likewise, red meat itself is not acidic; it just causes the stomach to release large quantities of stomach acid in order to break the meat down. The broken-down acidic-laden meat (chime) next enters the duodenum, which injects alkaline bile, but not enough to neutralize the overall acid level passing through. Hence, red meat drags higher levels of acid along with it into the intestines and therefore into the bloodstream. Once inside the bloodstream, meat metabolizes into acidic-leaning molecules further adding to the acid-forming effect throughout the body.

With this explanation of acidic- versus alkaline-forming foods in mind, the following chart illustrates the ranking of foods tied to acidity or alkalinity with food rankings further annotated based upon their sugar content (on a scale of 1-4, with 1 the least and 4 the most).

Acid (-) Versus Alkaline (+) Forming Food Rankings —

With Sugar-Laden Foods Italicized

Acid (-) Forming Foods

-4: *Pudding, jam, jelly, sugar, soda, ice cream,* beef, lobster, fried food, beer, antibiotics

-3: *Cranberry,* coffee, cottage cheese, pork, veal, mussels, chicken, corn, peanuts, carrots

-2: *Alcohol, white rice,* vanilla, black tea, balsamic vinegar, cheese, lamb, shell fish, beans, tomatoes

-1: *Honey, maple syrup, dried fruit,* cream, butter, yogurt, eggs, fish, brown rice, string beans, zucchini

Alkaline (+) Forming Foods

+1: *Oranges, grapes, blueberries, strawberries,* quinoa, wild rice, seeds, olive oil, brussel sprouts, beets, squash, lettuce

+2: *Pears, apples, cherries, peaches,* green tea, apple cider vinegar, almonds, potatoes, mushrooms, cauliflower, eggplant, lemon

+3: *Molasses, cantaloupe, honey dew,* soy sauce, cashews, peppers, garlic, asparagus, broccoli, endive, grapefruit, olives

+4: *Nectarines, raspberries, watermelon, tangerines, pineapple,* sea salt, mineral water, pumpkin seeds, seaweed, miso, sweet potatoes, limes

Please note that sea salt is a +4 and table salt is a -4. This dichotomy exists because sea salt is the very saline solution the body strives for, identical to the ocean. Conversely, when consuming table salt, the body tries to fix this "plain" salt invasion, wanting it to be sea salt. By robbing the blood of molecules to achieve this, the blood is left in an acidic state.

The Mayo Clinic claims that this differentiation between table salt and sea salt is unfounded as both substances are primarily the same — a whole lot of sodium nitrate. But that misses the point. The aspects that are different — the ninety trace elements in Himalayan sea salt, for instance — are the very elements the body craves. When these are missing, the body compensates by drawing internal molecules to the table salt to shore it up. Table salt is a free radical that steals molecules from the body.

Most of my comments regarding acidic- versus alkaline-forming foods comes from the research of ELIS/ACT Biotechnologies. Their PDF, "The Alkaline Way Guide," is available online.

One more comment about diet: a hamburger, fries, and a coke are about as bad as it gets. The hamburger causes acidity, and if charbroiled, comes with burnt-meat molecules that bind with sugar to increase glycation. The fries are carbs soon to be a sugar spike, cooked in oil and causing an intake of bad omega 6, which then neutralizes the body's good omega. The coke causes high acidity and sugar spikes.

Your poor liver cannot regulate all of this. Sugar and acid spikes occur in the bloodstream — and cancer rejoices.

Laura's diet started with less than 20 grams of carbohydrates per day causing her to become keytonic, hence dropping her weight to 113 pounds. Once there, she added chicken and fish every other day, keeping the carbohydrates low, but providing external fat to fuel the keytonic energy delivery mechanism that fed her healthy cells while isolating the cancer.

For a complete food listing see *"Green, Yellow & Red-Light Food Listings"* at the end of the appendices.

Defeating Breast Cancer

Chapter 11

Dietary Supplements

*B*esides depriving cancer, the cancer diet needs to fully provide food for all of the other cells of the body, and we achieve this through supplements. *Six* key dietary supplements surfaced: fatty acids, amino acids, CoQ10, the B vitamin family, vitamin C, and "vitamin" D. Vitamins A, E, and K tilt important as well, but these dwell in abundance inside green leafy plants, which Laura consumed daily.

Supplement #1— Fatty Acids—Omega 3

Omega-3 is referred to as a fatty acid (found in fats). Omega-3 supplements come from fish and krill oil, and most health professionals advocate supplements of omega-3 in your diet to counterbalance high omega-6 levels (omegas-3 and 6 need to balance each other out as this balance affects the previously mentioned BRCA 1 and 2 genes described below). Omega-3 bolsters the heart, tempers all sorts of mental issues like ADHA, and augments many other aspects of health, but for the purposes of this book, you should be aware of its role in preventing breast cancer.

Doctor Mercola explains:

"Two studies from 2002 explain how omega-3 can protect against breast cancer. BRCA1 (breast cancer gene 1) and BRCA2 (breast cancer gene 2) are two tumor-suppressor genes that, when functioning normally, help repair DNA damage, a process that also prevents tumor development. Omega-3 and omega-6 fats have been found to influence these two genes—omega-3 tends to reduce cancer cell growth, while highly processed and toxic omega-6 has been found to cause cancer growth.

Omega-6 excesses come mainly from certain cooking oils—vegetable, canola, and so on—and to temper this, you should switch to olive oil and butter. We use a unique omega-3 supplement that claims to be easily absorbed by the intestines.

Supplement #2—Amino Acids

The body comprises roughly 70 percent water, with the next largest substance, protein, at 20 percent of overall body weight. (*Protein* in biological speak means an organic molecule, not meat.) All of the structural aspects of cells and most of the chemical agents directed by cellular RNA comprise various configurations of protein.

Amino acids form the chemical building blocks the body uses to create these varied proteins. In chapter X, we described how consumed proteins of animals and plants are reduced to amino acids that the human body reassembles to make human specific proteins. Hence, you need an adequate and constant pool of amino acids running through your system for the full fuel requirements of normal cells.

As previously discussed, when we digest proteins such as meat or fish, the digestive track breaks down the source proteins into amino acids that are absorbed by the intestines and sent up to the liver for additional processing. Just as the body requires a persistent availability of oxygen supplied by the lungs, the liver releases the amino acids to the heart at a constant rate to be continuously available to all 100 trillion cells. The cells, in turn, convert the incoming amino acids into the protein required at the moment (not the exact protein found in the ingested chicken).

Although the liver does a good job in spreading out the delivery of amino acids to the body, it can only release as much as it is given, so …if you do not absorb enough amino acids because of a lack in your diet or to other absorption issues, then all 100 trillion cells become handicapped. This "starvation" phenomenon increases as you age, and so amino acid deficiency creeps up on you.

The major amino acids include: argintine, carnitine, glutamine, methionine, ornithine, and taurine. You should read up on each of these, and work with a nutrinionist to decipher which shortage is causing your specific symptoms. For example, the heart muscle particularly requires taurine. If you have heart issues, perhaps an uneven rhythm, you may have a taurine deficiency. A good cardiologist might want to try a very small dose to evaluate if it might bring any potential relief.

In the case of cancer, a debate rages over argintine, which affects the circulatory system by enabling blood flow and delivering greater levels of oxygen throughout the body. Proponents say that this boost of oxygen acts as a poison to the cancer tumors; detractors say that enhanced blood flow enhances the nutrient levels reaching the tumor. We added an argentine supplement to the plan as it is oxygen oriented, and anyway, we were already depriving cancer cells of sugars.

Another option we investigated but did not adopt is CAAT—Controlled Amino Acid Therapy. Here, those amino acids believed to provide cancer cells with nutrition are eliminated while other amino acids that boost the immune system are added. This treatment includes a very specific daily diet. The researchers involved claim CAAT works faster to shrink tumors than basic sugar deprivation.

Supplement #3—Coenzyme 10 (CoQ10)

The literature claims that our little friends, the mitochondria, directly access CoQ10 and that the little buggers need it to do their job. *CoQ10* is a coenzyme found in many foods and assembled by the liver. People who take CoQ10 have more vitality, and so I added a mild dose of CoQ10 to the self-healing plan once I thought Laura's cells had been detoxified and were ready to go.

The Mayo Clinic says this about CoQ10:

"CoQ10 levels decrease with age and may be low in people with cancer, certain genetic disorders, diabetes, heart conditions, HIV/AIDS, muscular dystrophy, and Parkinson's disease. Some prescription drugs may also lower CoQ10 levels. CoQ10 in the body can be increased by taking CoQ10 supplements."

Later, Doctor Bard (The New York City doctor who administered the 3-D sonogram) added his own CoQ10 formula to the plan, which had more potency.

Supplement #4 — The Vitamin B Family

The vitamin B family contains eight varieties of B vitamins including the special B12 vitamin that is usually deficient in most of us. Apparently, these variants of vitamin B, each in its own way, help the liver to further break down digested food so that cells can absorb the nutrients; plus, vitamin B provides nutrients to the various elements of the nervous system (described further in the "Loose Ends" chapter).

Consumers can find vitamin B complex supplements anywhere, and you should take a modest dose as part of the self-healing plan. Based upon blood nutrition tests, a special B12/folic acid supplement might be a good idea as well.

When we added argentine to the plan, it included the B family, and we used this approach rather than a strict B supplement.

Supplement #5 — Vitamin C

Let's look at vitamin C's important attributes.

First, your body does not produce or store vitamin C. It is ingested, "water-soluble," floating through the bloodstream, continually purged by the kidneys; so new vitamin C is needed each day.

Second, vitamin C is a "reducing agent," meaning it readily donates electrons to "free radical" molecules thereby neutralizing (reducing) these scavengers.

Third, vitamin C is a great antioxidant. It provides a molecular skin that protects cell walls from being exposed to oxygen. It also protects from oxidation the body's supply of fats, proteins, and vitamins that are floating around in the bloodstream..

Fourth, it is required to make the previously discussed collagen (the body's bungee cords).

Nevertheless, the body can only absorb around 500 mg of vitamin C at a time, and mega-doses disrupt various systems in the body, such as the digestive track and your sleep, while also making the kidneys work overtime. The Mayo Clinic recommends 2,000 units a day, but many would double this when your system is under attack by a virus as long as it is spread out over the twenty-four-hour cycle.

Laura (and I) stayed with moderate doses of vitamin C and never caught a cold. The 1,000 unit Emergen-C product was our weapon of choice as it delivers vitamin C as well as electrolytes. Never getting a cold gave me confidence that our cells were well protected against viral attack.

A vitamin C controversy: For thirty years, I've heard claims that cancer thrives in a vitamin C-rich environment. Looking into this, all I found was that vitamin C blunts the effect of certain chemo treatments. Part of the chemo effect is to expose the tumor to oxygen, and vitamin C shields the tumor from oxygen because it is an antioxidant. But this chemo-specific effect is very different from cancer actually thriving on vitamin C. It thrives on sugar.

Supplement #6 — "Vitamin" D

Notice the quotation marks around the word "vitamin." This is because "vitamin" D is not really a vitamin; it is a hormonal steroid.

Vitamins like the Bs and C are outside molecules supplied from food used to build cells, create antioxidants, and to metabolize nutrients; vitamins are *externally* supplied "ingredients," if you will. Hormonal steroids, on the other hand, are *internally* created by the body to cause behavioral responses in cells such as telling the brain you are hungry; they are "cellular traffic cops" if you will. D is one of these internally made steroid molecules though most people still incorrectly refer to D as an ingested vitamin rather than as a sunlight-triggered chemical formation in the skin.

D works as a *systemic steroid* meaning that it affects every cell in the body working to keep the specialized cell types on course as they divide, for example, making sure dividing lung cells produce lung cells, hair cells produce hair cells, and so on. The various cell types all have the same set of 20,000 chromosomes. Cells specialize through the already mentioned switch settings governing the chromosomes. A lung cell has the same genes as a liver cell, but specific gene switch settings make it a liver cell.

Stem cells, the exception, start neutral, and have no switches turned off or on. For example, when a stem cell morphs into a muscle cell, it copies the switch settings of a muscle cell.

D is a "cheerleader-like" stimulant telling the genes to stay switched. All kinds of D receptors reside inside the cell waiting to talk to D so genes can stay reassured as to their proper setting. When cells are not "reassured," they become "lost" and malfunction, probably resulting in everything from depression to breast cancer to autism. For instance, according to Doctor Mercola, a strong link exists between D and autism as follows:

"In more recent years, rampant vitamin D deficiency has been linked to a proportionate jump in autism. While the connection may not be obvious, it's important to realize that vitamin D receptors appear in a wide variety of brain tissue during early fetal development, and activated vitamin D receptors increase nerve growth in your brain."

Researchers have also located metabolic pathways for vitamin D in the hippocampus and cerebellum of the brain, areas that are involved in planning, processing information, and the formation of new memories. The National Institutes of Mental Health concluded that it is *vital* that an expectant mother get enough vitamin D while pregnant for the baby's brain to develop properly.

My take on autism is different, though the lack of D can be a factor in neurons not being created properly. If D were the main driver, autism would have been around forever. Instead, I propose a new phenomenon inserted into the environment around thirty years ago as the trigger of autism: pesticide-coated seeds.

Rather than spraying growing plants from above via plane as was done in the past, the seed itself is now sprayed and coated with pesticides so that the germinating plant carries the poison inside of it. Pesticide poisons are formulated to disrupt the nervous system of the insects feeding off the plant. This is why bees get lost trying to find their hive after ingesting pesticide-laden pollen. With modern-day mothers eating food derived from such plants, enough nerve-debilitating toxins reach the fetus, and if the mother also lacks in D, the neurons cannot develop fully.

OK, back to "D"

The body creates D mainly from sunlight that penetrates your skin. But many people today do not get enough sunlight and hence not enough D. This deficiency descends to every cell in the body, with specialized cells like brain or breast cells negatively affected by a lack of D in their own specific "gene-switch-confused" manner.

A nutrient blood test can measure your D, and if you are found deficient, your diet specialist can recommend a supplement dosage. By the way, when under mental stress or exertion, the brain draws down huge quantities of D, so your standing D level needs a built-in reserve.

A report in the *Journal of Neurology* by a Doctor Llewellyn cites that the risk of dementia dramatically increases as one's level of D decreases (though I proscribe the pesticide cause here as well). Likewise, the *British Medical Journal* published findings that for those with a history of breast cancer, lack of D increased the chance of getting cancer by 70 percent. "D" is a must-have supplement that affects everything, ESPECIALLY IF THE CELL HAS BEEN WEAKENED BY A TOXIN.

Overall, with D and the other supplements, the goal remains to give the cells a supply boost so that they can execute their functions more vigorously including augmenting internal cell defenses against viruses and providing nutrients for immune system cells to fight the good fight against viruses and cancer occurrences.

Note, in 2019, as I prepared this edition for publication, Doctor Bronstein published an in depth analysis on Vitamin E, and how it strengthens cell walls against things like viruses and oxidants. Please consider adding some E, along with the green leafy plants that naturally supply it. Take your supplements!

Next, boosting the immune system.

Part V

Boosting the Body

Chapter 12

Boosting the Immune System

*B*ecause Laura started strong right away with the cleansing and diet tactics, she fundamentally established the pillars of her plan by Week 4. Now we wanted to strengthen the resolve of her immune system. We could surely consider *many* approaches to bolster this vast military operation. After a lot of reading, it came down to two supplements: *red Reishi mushroom extract* and *beta-glucan*. But to appreciate these, we must first peek into the fundamentals of the immune system. Here goes.

Offense and Defense

The functions of the body exist as two main camps: offense and defense.

The offense camp includes the nourishment and respiratory functions — eating, breathing, digestion, vascular delivery, liver and kidney filtering, and waste disposal. These functions bring in and distribute minerals, vitamins, fats, sugars, amino acids, proteins, and oxygen to each of the trillions of cells in the body. Once the body delivers these, the biochemistry inside each cell (including the aerobic actions of the mitochondria described later) blends resources to fuel the cells' existence. Mathematically, I cannot say how many simultaneous offensive cellular-level chemical events occur within our gigantic life systems, but I can try.

We estimate that each of our bodies possesses 100 trillion cells, and within each cell, a million molecular events might occur at any given moment: that's 100 trillion cells multiplied by one million molecular events in concurrent action (let's call it … "a gazillion"). Electric energy packets manufactured by the cell's mitochondria propel these molecular actions (as promised, more to come on this). This, then constitutes the offensive side of the body, the camp driving life forward.

The Defensive Camp

The *immune system defense camp* comprises the second camp, and the body charges it with "watching the back" of the entire offensive operation. The "all-defense, all-the-time" immune system stands as quite an operation in its own right, and rightfully so! At every moment, millions of "microbes" (viruses, bacteria, fungi, parasites) as well as *toxins* (lead, mercury, pesticides, carbon monoxide, etc.) enter your body. As is often said in sports, "Defense often trumps offense."

Before going into some further detail on how the defensive immune system works, just consider what could go wrong with the offensive side of the body if the defensive side lets the invaders get the upper hand. The result? Death via infection regardless of whether viral, bacterial, fungi, parasites, or toxic agents drive that infection. This need for a massive defense against a mathematically unfathomable attack by foreign enemies makes boosting the immune system a mandatory strategy toward keeping cancer in check.

Let's look in some detail at how the immune system works.

Immune System Mechanics 101

The immune system comprises an entire set of specialized cells and protein molecules geared to detect foreign agents and kill them ASAP. These forces can be divided into various specialized units, which through chemical signaling among themselves, formulate an overall defensive shield for the body. I'll provide a high-altitude view of what's going on in the trenches, inside each of these specialty camps in the following sections.

Antibodies — The Searchers: White blood cells secrete these proteins (*antibodies* are nonliving proteins) which, like snowflakes, come in millions of shapes and sizes. They flow through the body and bump into things, looking for "foreigners" (the aforementioned viruses, bacteria, fungi, and parasites).

Each foreigner bears a unique chemical appendage on its surface (think of it as a "lock"). To pick this lock, the millions of unique "antibody" proteins floating around represent potential "keys" to that lock. If an antibody's molecular key happens to line up with the foreigner's lock, then they bind. Scientific language refers to these chemical structures (the "locks" and the "keys") as *receptors*.

Once a match occurs between the respective receptors, the antibody scout (which carries only a whistle and not a loaded gun) releases another chemical to warn the rest of the immune system that *a bad guy has been identified – backup is needed.* Backup primarily comes in the form of gun-carrying T-cells, natural killer cells, macrophages, and neutrophils.

When none of the millions of antibody receptors in circulation match up with the foreigner's receptor, the foreigner runs wild, undetected, proliferating for days within the body. The white blood cells must somehow create a new antibody protein whose receptor *does* match the foreigner's receptor; otherwise, the infection will remain undetected and will take over and kill the body one cell at a time.

Sometimes, a key cannot be found and the invader wins killing the host (that's you) – this happens with viruses such as Ebola or viral pneumonia. But most of the time, the attacking virus is sought out, marked, and assaulted by various immune agents as follows:

B-Cells – The Librarians: After all the effort taken to find a match between the receptor surface of an antibody protein and the receptor surface of a foreigner, the immune system wants to file the new finding away for future reference. This way, if the foreigner ever comes back, the immune system can forego all of this searching and quickly roll out the exact antibody needed to match up with the foreigner to quickly identify the foreigner for what it is – a foreigner.

This filing system of foreigners and their receptor layouts is the job of B-cells. B-cells circle around the blood system looking for antibodies already attached to foreigners, antibodies currently sending out SOSs. The B-cell copies down all of this valuable receptor data for posterity.

When a B-cell cannot find work — there are no antibodies SOS-ing for help — it dies, and your bone marrow releases new B-cells to start the journey all over again. When a B-cell *does* get work, it imprints the receptor layout of the foreign antigen onto itself, and rather than die, the enlightened B-cell proliferates (divides). Thereafter, it secretes antibodies that fit those specific foreign receptors so that future encounters with that same foreign antigen are quickly deciphered. Go, B-cells!

BTW, scientifically, medical papers, should you dare to read them, refer to these foreigners as *antigens.*

That's why it seems that you don't usually catch the same flu strain twice (actually, you *do* catch it again, but B-cells quickly detect it). Go B-cells again!

This librarian role of B-cells brings up the topic of vaccines. *Vaccines* proactively allow the body to find and stow the antibody key to a particular disease within our B-cell library. A *vaccine* contains a chemical fingerprint of a disease-causing microorganism made from weakened or killed forms of the microbe, its toxins, or one of its surface proteins. The injected fingerprint agent stimulates the body's immune system to find an antibody that will mark the agent as a threat, and then keep a B-cell record of it. Going forward, the immune system can more easily recognize and destroy any of these microorganisms that it later encounters.

It is often said, "Without vaccines, mass infections of whole populations would take place."

Yet, there is controversy concerning vaccines as many parents have had their children become feverishly ill upon being vaccinated and later found their child's personality or mental abilities permanently altered. According to Doctor

Bronstein, "The vast majority of flu vaccines are preserved with a mercury compound called thimerosal. Many vaccines contain other toxic additives such as the carcinogen formaldehyde." Hmmm…

T-Cells — The Foot Soldiers: Once antibodies "smoke out" the antigens (foreigners), T-cells actually kill foreign antigens. Overall, we refer to them as T-cells because the stem cells they originate from change into immune system cells inside the thymus (T) gland in the neck. (As a footnote: An example of the aging process provides that the thymus gland produces 3 percent fewer T-cells per year once we enter middle age. Yikes, we need all of the T-cells we can get if we are to live forever.)

Unfortunately, the thymus gland often produces imperfect T-cells that cannot distinguish between normal and foreign cells (they are very bad cops). These dangerous T-cells are usually killed off themselves; if not, they aggressively go after normal cells, hence the "autoimmune" diseases of Lupus and AIDS. Lupus malfunctions remain a mystery. AIDS, however, is a virus (viruses again!) that has co-opted the T-cells.

Natural Killer (NK) Cells — Special Forces: NK Cells are another type of *white blood cell* (cells that come directly from the bone marrow, not matured by the thalamus gland) that *specialize in hunting tumor cells and viruses* (the same thing really if you accept my virus theory of cancer).

Unlike T-cells, which need antibodies to first flag down the foreign antigens, NK cells "frisk" encountered suspects to find out if the entity carries a "self" marker (a chemical form of proper ID). Should the NK cells find no evidence of self-marking, they then bore holes in the foreign entity filling it with poisons like oxygen (a nasty business).

Monocytes and Macrophages – The Mop-Up Squad: These long-living (two months) cells seek out and destroy dying or infected cells and other "debris" to keep the body clean, thus fostering healing. A "baby" monocyte arrives as a junior version of the ultimate macrophage cell just coming out of "boot camp" (the *bone marrow* is the boot camp), so to speak. But when other immune cells finally call them into action, the immature monocytes quickly morph into various macrophage forms, now essentially "special ops" cells that respond to different tissue type malfunctions throughout the body.

Besides mopping up dying cells, cancer cells, and foreign invaders, the mature macrophages biochemically direct other immune cells through receptor signals when the "crime site" requires more work.

When out of work, the macrophage specialists simply "hang out" in nearby barracks (usually in connecting bone joints) and await the next call of duty.

I am not making this up!

Neutrophil – The First Responders: Each day, the bone marrow releases 100 billion neutrophil immune system cells into the bloodstream. They move throughout the body, do their job, and then die within hours of being deployed. Their job: penetrate every nook and cranny of the body at the capillary level and lie in wait for chemical "SOS" signals — called *chemo taxis* — secreted by any nearby injured or infected cells asking for immediate help.

Neutrophil cells come running and cause inflammation and puss in the infected area effectively "holding the fort" until the "big guy" white blood cells can come in to do the heavy lifting. Once the neutrophil's short, one-hour life ends after having not found anything, a big macrophage scavenger cell eliminates the tiny neutrophil scout (remember, "No good deed goes unpunished").

Again, I am not making this stuff up.

The preceding description provides a flavor of the enormous moment-by-moment, chemically induced operation of the immune system, which is orchestrated using gazillions of cell and protein receptor matchups to spur further chemical releases that spur further events—all rigged to kill real foreigners such as bacteria, viruses, fungi, and parasites, and to kill rogue cells that have turned cancerous.

So given all of the effort put forward by the immune system on your behalf, the only thing you might want to add is the question:

What can I do to help?

Research turned up the following.

Beta-Glucans

Glucans—Glucans, a nutritional molecule that you get from various foods including grains and mushrooms, appear to help on two fronts—reducing high cholesterol and boosting the immune system. We like both of these.

On the cholesterol-benefit side, the fibrous nature of glucans helps inside the digestive tract. Glucan molecules bind with excess cholesterol molecules creating an inert substance that the body purges, thankfully, rather than absorbs. Hence, the following quote from the European Food Information Council:

"*Beta-glucan*, a type of dietary fiber found in abundance in oats, has been recognized as having blood cholesterol-lowering properties. A major proposed mechanism is that dietary oat beta-glucan forms a viscous layer in the small intestine. The viscous layer attenuates the intestinal uptake of dietary cholesterol as well as the reabsorption of bile acids (which the body makes from cholesterol). In response, the body draws upon the pool of circulating cholesterol to produce new bile acids. Lower uptake of cholesterol from the gut combined with more bodily cholesterol used for bile acid production results in reduced levels of cholesterol circulating in the blood."

On the immune-system-benefit side, glucan acts as an *immunomodulation* agent (I often wonder who made this word up), meaning that it heightens the activity of the immune system. The immune attack cells grow more aggressive, and communication among the specialized immune cells becomes more emphatic not unlike a basketball team suddenly shifting into "domination mode" on the court. To give you a flavor of scientific writing, consider a few sentences from this research report on beta-glucans from the 2009 *Journal Of Hematology & Oncology*:

"Glucans act on several immune receptors including Dectin-1, complement receptor (CR3), and TLR-2/6 and trigger a group of immune cells including macrophages, neutrophils, monocytes, and natural killer cells. Glucans are captured by the macrophages via the Dectin-1 receptor with or without TLR-2/6. The large glucan molecules are then internalized and fragmented into smaller-sized glucan fragments within the macrophages. They are carried to the marrow and endothelial reticular system and subsequently released. These small glucan fragments are eventually taken up by the circulating granulocytes, monocytes, or macrophages via the complement receptor (CR)-3. The immune response will then be turned on; one of the actions is the phagocytosis of the monoclonal-antibody-tagged tumor cells."

This last, perhaps indecipherable sentence simply means that tumor cells tagged by antibodies as "foreign" suddenly appear visible to the immune cells, which can now devour (the process is called *phagocytosis)* the tumor. I keep wondering: How do young premed people memorize these incoherent descriptions?

Because glucan comes into the bloodstream through digestion, we can easily supplement it by taking glucan-extract pills. The body uses what it wants, so having elevated levels of glucan moving through the small intestine cannot hurt; this simply ensures the continuous presence of an ample level to fortify each of the billions of immune cells the bone marrow and the thymus gland deploy each hour. Take glucans!

Red Reishi Mushrooms

There is a common understanding among people that mushrooms are special though few know why this might be so. The world offers many varieties of mushrooms, and many offer valuable nutrients not readily found elsewhere. But the red Reishi mushroom sits atop the heap with its various "active agents," molecules that dramatically affect cells in the human body including offering its own unique glucan molecule.

Very notable: Red Reishi pushes immune system cells to attack "impenetrable" tumors, and not just "tiny" viruses and bacteria. Scientifically, I do not know why this is so, but many, many health practitioners claim that it is true.

Where are the young, driven PhD candidates on this topic?

In Eastern medicine for two thousand years, doctors who cared for Oriental royal families prescribed red Reishi, which was at first rare and difficult to gather as it only grew in a natural setting on certain decaying tree trunks. But recently, the Japanese finally found a way to cultivate it in greenhouses with its extracts now available in pill form (thank you, Japan). Other Reishi species exist, but the red ones remain the cat's meow as far as the immune system goes. Some also use red Reishi for high blood pressure and other ailments. *Natural News* describes Reishi as follows:

"Research shows that the polysaccharide beta-1,3-D-glucan in Reishi boosts the immune system by raising the amount of macrophages and T-cells. This immune-boosting action works wonders in the prevention and treatment of cancer. In addition to boosting immune system numbers, the glucan in Reishi helps immune cells bind to tumor cells. Another substance in Reishi, called *canthaxanthin*, slows down the growth of tumors. It directly reduces the number of cancerous cells making it easier for T-cells and macrophages to rid the body of them. Research and traditional medicinal usage of Reishi to fight cancer is so positive that the Japanese government officially recognizes it as a cancer treatment."

I find that paragraph about as lucid a medical science paragraph as you might find while researching these sorts of things, and so I included it here. Most scientific writing contains so many Greek and Latin words framed in obtuse medical jargon that you have little or no chance of understanding them unless you devote days on end to solving the word puzzles and obtuse content and try to put it in context. Still, I recommend that you dig into medical studies on all kinds of things and grow accustomed to the babble! Deciphering medical babble changes your mind from that of a passive accepter of the authority of medical intervention to an active prospector of new knowledge, a mind-set that dovetails beautifully with the self-healing plan.

Other research uncovered the following about immune cells.

Immune System Breakdowns — Crone's Disease

Crone's disease, named after Dr. Crone who first described the condition in the early 1900s, occurs when your immune system mistakenly attacks good bacteria in your intestines creating vast amounts of inflammation both in the intestines and throughout the whole body. Why the immune system is fixated on killing the good digestive bacteria is unknown.

A possible construct to explain Crone's comes back to viruses. In this theory (my theory), the viruses in question do not invade the body's cells but instead infect the trillions of bacteria living symbiotically inside of your digestive track. The infected bacteria nevertheless attract bodily immune scouts looking for foreigners (antigens), but instead of creating antibodies identifying the virus, the immune cells "mark" the sickly bacteria as the problem.

Once catalogued as trouble by the librarian B cells, the immune attack cells target the innocent bacteria in the intestines filling the intestines with inflammation in an attempt to stem the "perceived" enemy. If B cells indeed permanently mark the good bacteria for execution— allowing the Crone's condition to cycle for decades until death—the solution to Crone's lies in removing incorrect "antigen" designations within B cells. Until B cell rehabilitation is deciphered, Crone's sufferers should calm down the immune system by detoxing and should chip away at inflammation deposits via enzymes that break down inflammation (described in chapter 18).

Body Heat

One other note on the immune system: It becomes more active when body temperatures rise (fever). One of the reasons Laura took a hot bath each evening was to switch her system to the restful sleep state where the immune system is most active, but the corollary reason was to raise her temperature, even slightly, to further encourage immune cells.

One final note on the immune system.

T-Cell Manipulation

One of the difficulties in fighting cancer solely using your own immune system is that the immune system cells recognize cancer cells as a natural part of the body. Cancer cells are not seen and attacked the way viruses, bacteria, fungi, and parasites are. CBD oil, mentioned earlier, helps to make cancer more visible by sticking to the cancer cell walls making them look somewhat foreign. And while the CBD tactic helps by illuminating the cancer cells, a reciprocal tactic, called cimetric antigen receptor (CAR) T-cells, is in the works that make the immune cells more capable of finding the diseased cells as follows.

Researchers have found a way to reconfigure your T-cell gene switches so that T-Cell "search" receptors more closely pair up with the unique receptors sitting on cancer cell walls. This plan first harvests T-cells from the patient, which are then genetically manipulated and allowed to multiply into the billions of cells. These reconfigured T-cells are then infused back into the patient where they quickly hook up with cancer counterparts killing the cancer in the same manner immune cells kill all foreigners.

So far, this immune system empowerment plan is used for blood cancers, like leukemia, but it should work for others as well. But just keep in mind that the core manner for controlling cancer remains not to feed it. Starve the cancer and then send in the troops!

Chapter 13

Boosting Energy

*C*ommon sense dictates that you benefit from as much energy as you can muster during normal times, and that energy grows even more valuable when trying to put cancer back into its box. "Energy," however, is just a word, and so this chapter first fleshes out what we mean by "energy" and then elaborates on what to do about it in the context of the self-healing plan.

What *Is* Energy?

Mankind *barely* understands energy. Yes, we know how to harness it by burning wood in a fireplace or by creating vast electrical charges in power plants, but that does not mean we understand energy any more than we understand matter. Einstein advanced our understanding by *imagining* that energy and matter cannot be destroyed, just exchanged, and that the relationship between energy and matter is $E=MC^2$. Still, Albert never said what matter and energy *are*; he just knew how to measure them.

But for sure, it seems certain that when we live, much of this "mysterious" energy resides in our bodies. And, as stated in an earlier chapter, once the energy ends, the 100-trillion biochemical cell factories pumping away inside each of us grind to a halt. And we die. So, it behooves us to understand the role of energy in our health, especially if cancer is on the march inside of our bodies. But before we talk health, let's talk physics for a brief moment.

Various types of energies employ things called *subatomic particles* to cause their energy "results." *Photons*, for example, are *electromagnetic energy* particles that transport light energy. A photon has no weight; it is pure energy. For example, plants capture photons from the sun to fuel photosynthesis.

Electrons are negatively "charged" non-mass particles (whatever that really means) pulled toward the positively "charged" protons inside atoms' nuclei. Somehow, electrons can also assemble *en masse* outside of proton influences, such as in the case of lightning bolts or in the form of *electric energy* moving through our power grids

PS: I grew up with practicing electrical engineers of the highest rank, the builders of power plants, and none of these gurus could explain any of this. Like Einstein, they knew how to measure electrical phenomenon with equations, but they never could explain the electrical entity itself.

Next, consider subatomic *nuclear energy* particles called *bosons* that hold atoms together. (Hey, who knew that atoms needed help?) Then envision subatomic *gravitational energy* particles that draw discrete bodies together (such as Earth and the moon), effectively holding the moon and us humans to Earth. No one has isolated or measured these particles, but we already refer to them as *gravitons*. I can only imagine the endless exchange of weightless graviton particles between Earth and our feet, like a gravitational river running all day long! Yet another subatomic particle, *phonons,* are vibrating particles that create a wave effect in air or water. Long-wavelength phonons give rise to *sound.* Shorter wavelength, higher-frequency phonons give rise to *heat.*

And so, every energy force has its particle facilitator, connecting related entities, and, at every given moment, all of these energy forces and their entire infinitesimal particle exchanges operate according to some grand scheme scientists have yet to discover. This gigantic, interactive energy dynamic proves universally true for stagnant piles of dust, for rocks, oceans, the stars, and our human bodies.

Human bodies? We are surely different from rocks, aren't we?

Life energy – a force already spoken of in earlier chapters – binds all of these disparate forces together into a coherent living system. Yet, as with gravity, we can currently only observe life energy, and as with gravity, we have not yet isolated its particles. We gauged life energy, first in ancient Asian cultures and now in the West, as a network of meridians strung throughout the body. Moreover, you can increase your flow of life energy as a boost to your good health.

In a nutshell, we have observed that where life energy stands strong, you are near invincible; where life energy sags weakly, the body loses resolve and grows ill. And when life energy leaves the body, the cells die, soon returning to dust. All of this energy stuff—life, gravity, nuclear, light, and heat, and so on—plays out inside the biological world.

I have much more to say about life energy later. But first a look, finally, at its surrogates, the precious mitochondria.

Mitochondria—Biological Energy

Now, we'll visit one of the most amazing things I discovered through my recent research: a subspecies called *mitochondria* that lives inside our cells. As I learned more about this, I would mention the word *mitochondria* to friends, and it surprised me that they all knew mitochondria as "the cell's energy power center," drawing comparisons to a Duracell AAA battery. But that catchphrase proved *all* they knew about the little buggers.

For example, the theory holds that these mitochondria really exist as a form of bacteria that has lived symbiotically inside our cells...forever. *Symbiotically* in this case means that mitochondria have struck a deal with our cells: They make energy packets used by the cell, and in return, the mitochondria get to tap into all those juicy nutrients arriving from the cell's outer membrane. Then I learned that mitochondria have their own DNA, meaning that they can reproduce on their own.

I was flabbergasted.

The mitochondria's DNA stands separate from a cell's big DNA library, which resides inside the cell's nucleus membrane. Mitochondria have a relatively short DNA strand as the mitochondria only do a few things, such as churn molecules to cause energy releases and divide and multiply to meet the cell's need for energy. (They apparently spin at an amazing 1,000 RPM, revolutions per minute, pace.)

The kicker: Hundreds up to thousands of these autonomous mitochondria "things" live inside every cell of the body—that's 100 trillion human cells multiplied by thousands of mitochondria per cell. Gazillions of mitochondria "agents" live within us, and they are all busy-as-bees making "energy." This is a truly amazing phenomenon for anyone such as me to contemplate as I thought, "I was I, and only I!" Now I find that I am I…and a gazillion little buddies! (Note: Heart and neuron cells have the most mitochondria, as these cells are in high gear 24/7. Bone cells, on the other hand, might have only a handful.)

Apparently, these mitochondria maniacs spin like turbines, day and night, combining phosphates, oxygen, and other molecules, releasing some sort of usable energy packets that propel the endless biochemical activities of the cell.

The energy generated: electrical charges housed in a molecule called *ATP*, an organic battery that holds an extra electron, which when released powers the chemical processes inside the cell. I cannot grasp what that actually means though it is written about in countless medical papers.

But our understanding, as shallow as it is, stops here, as no one can describe how this ethereal energy animates the millions of moving chemical interactions happening within the cell. Though obviously at the edge of knowledge, by grasping the proliferation of mitochondria throughout the body, we can nevertheless grasp the dimension of the vast energy potential of the body. Its energy output is nearly endless, a perpetual and demanding furnace, burning the nutrients, oxygen, and enzymes that keep us alive one moment at a time.

By the way, before we get to the even more important stuff, I learned that you inherit your mitochondria from the unfertilized egg supplied by your mother. We refer to mitochondrial DNA as mtDNA and use it in tracking genealogies going all the way back to "Eve." I wonder, are some people born with better mitochondria than others? Someone could earn a PhD on this topic alone!

But ponder the bigger questions: What keeps trillions upon trillions of mitochondria spinning? What keeps them working so hard, night and day, cellular division after cellular division, across an entire human lifetime? And why do they all stop spinning at once when we die?

I cannot prove it, but I believe mitochondria—like from a gruff Newark, New Jersey airport cop—get the "keep moving" impulse from the life energy network pulsating through the body. I theorize that if the life energy switch is "on," then all systems are "go." Keep moving! Turn the switch "off," and every mitochondrial light attached to the grid goes out, a permanent power outage.

Despite biology's impressive known and endless unknowns of mitochondria, I felt that Laura and I ought to help the little buggers out if we could. After all, they remain totally loyal to us on a 24/7 basis, and, more important, we apparently (and desperately) need them as they could simply kill us should they decide to go on strike.

Physical Therapy, Supplements, and Double Helix Water

To tend to the wants and desires of these mysterious yet noble mitochondria, Laura and I decided to use physical therapy, nutritional supplements (discussed in chapter 11), and a special type of water called *double helix water* to win them over; we offered them the kitchen sink, if you will. I talk about physical therapy and double helix water in the following sections.

Physical Therapy—As previously discussed, Laura met with Stephen Karpenko, a kinseologist on a weekly basis. His job? To determine if any weak energy flows existed in her meridians, and if so, to take corrective action through *manipulation* (chiropractic adjustment), *stimulation* (acupuncture), or through strengthening (exercising areas of physiological tissue weakness). In the first year, Laura received kinesiologist evaluation and treatment thirty times. Given the discussion above on energy and health, these weekly (and later bimonthly) macrolevel tune-ups remain essential; we want *all* of the lights on *all* of the time.

Let's step back. Earlier in the book, I mentioned the thermography heat and cold exam.

They found two points of "trauma" that bookended a specific meridian that runs through Laura's right breast, exactly where the two cancer tumors lined up. The assumption that this "compromised" meridian had not operated properly for an extended period of time implies the following:

Cells along the meridian had long received weak life energy encouragement from the meridian grid. This, in turn, affected each cell's mitochondria energy output, which implicitly lowered each cell's ability to fight off outside viruses.

Assuming lower levels of energy prevailed, the thinking is that viruses furiously and continuously bombard outer membrane cell walls trying to get in, and that each cell needs to drive millions of internal "protein antibody and protein crusher molecules" prowling inside to thwart the penetrating invaders. GEEZ!

Each of these operating proteins, though needs ample energy to fulfill its role, or as the decidedly politically incorrect saying goes from our baby boomer 1950s childhood: "No ticky, no laundry."

The "low energy" condition similarly affects the immune cells deployed to patrol the breast meridian area; they become sluggish in prosecuting any cancer cells they encounter.

The maxim: *Impeded life energy leads to illness.* The lightbulbs may be on, but they glow very dimly. The kinesiologist worked to get these lights to once again burn brightly.

So, you might ask, what else could possibly remain to boost energy levels (besides boosting oxygen, described later)?

The answer: water.

"Double Helix Water" proved the most far-out finding of my research, but *don't* dismiss it! Here goes...

Double Helix Water — Double helix water is a physical state of the H2O water molecule. The three states of H2O

---

we know include: ice (solid), water (liquid), and vapor (gas, "steam"), but a fourth state exists. The fourth state remains an H2O molecule, but the atoms are packed very tightly together, even more so than when in the ice state (generally as molecules cool, their atomic particles move closer together). Double helix water molecules, however, already exist extremely packed together, even when they are in water of 100 to 200 degrees Fahrenheit. Rather than through temperature, double helix water molecules bind tighter due to extraordinary electrical charges.

OK, so where does this special molecule take us in the discussion of life energy?

As stated earlier, our bodies are as much as 70 percent water, which amounts to around 100 trillion cells to the "unimaginable" power in water molecules sitting inside all of us, a quantity we cannot possibly fathom. The double helix water molecule exists among these, spread evenly throughout the body, with each double helix molecule carrying a supercharge of electricity.

I believe that collectively, the double helix water charges combine to form the meridian grid within the body, exchanging immense quantities of subatomic "charge" particles to cause the effect we call *life energy.*

In the laboratory, scientists have found ways to isolate and concentrate the double helix water molecules. When put into close proximity, these molecules draw each other closer and — get this — take on the shape of a double-helix DNA strand, forming the spiraling ladder with water molecules rather than genes. These electrically charged H2O molecules, found in every glass of water and in every ocean, apparently seek to organize matter across other energy fields (gravity, nuclear, electromagnetic, etc.) into the form of life's core helix structure.

This did it for me, as I have been 100 percent sure of life energy's existence for years having witnessed four births and five deaths but could never envision a particle exchange framework to hang the concept onto the way all other energy fields function. Unlike all of the drugs doctors prescribe that are inherently alien to our DNA libraries, water, including the double helix molecules, is inherently natural fitting in nicely with the overall DNA program. By ingesting concentrated vials of double helix water, you might increase the cellular energy above the norm for, say, a fifty-year-old person.

And so, upon understanding the attributes of double helix water molecules, I contacted the scientists in California working with double helix water and purchased some in order to boost the life energy current flowing through Laura's body.

The goal: *Keep all of her cells on their collective toes by keeping the mitochondrial lightbulbs burning as brightly as they wanted.*

Just to finish, a way to understand the life energy grid is the following: The meridian system already exists in an unfertilized human egg, a circle of energy bands inside the dish-like egg.

Upon fertilization, the egg splits. The split points become the mouth and anus ends of the torso, and the main meridians now run up and down the torso in this vertical manner. As the limbs develop, other horizontal meridians branch off to pulsate into these developing peripheral appendages, and so on.

But more, if this all proves true, then double helix water and the helix form it strives for may explain the backbone of all life on Earth (another prospective PhD paper). But one more energy management topic remains: sleep!

Sleep

Yes, we desire top-of-the-line, clean energy flowing among the cells, but we want the cells to rest and repair themselves as well. Therefore, we must understand *sleep,* a key element in the self-healing plan.

The nervous system possesses two basic states, *active awake* and *restful sleep* – the middle ground: insomnia and anxiety.

Situations can heighten the active awake state quite easily to what's called "fight or flight" levels based on what transpires during the day.

Days where every moment counts, where you find yourself driven, where you encounter threats or trouble, move you further out on the active awake spectrum toward "fight or flight."

We also call this "stress."

To cope with stress, your energy supply "revs" up so that you can ultimately bull yourself through the day. However, this approach does not bode well when trying to kill cancer.

When the system reaches high alert, it focuses energy toward the big fights taking place outside the body, reducing the energy available for the fights going on inside the body.

For example, when under stress, the adrenal gland releases a steroid hormone called *cortisol* to increase sugar and ultimately to suppress the immune system.

When fighting cancer, both of these outcomes are *bad*, and you should shield yourself from as much outside stress as possible to keep energy focused internally (*easier said than done*, I know, but a key factor nonetheless).

Cortisol is important. For a twenty-year-old soldier at war, *cortisol* is a good thing as it focuses the whole body and mind on the intensity of battle while telling the immune system to "stand down," at least "for now." But as one ages, the body's ability to deal with "fight or flight" intensity diminishes, yet the release of cortisol during moments of stress stays as constant at age fifty as when you were just twenty years old. Ultimately, with age, intense cortisol releases become problematic for many. Indeed, people with heart issues have most heart attacks and strokes within a two-hour window of instances of stress where copious amounts of cortisol remain in the system.

If you have cancer, you must reduce the triggers for stress and those moments when cortisol is released with all of the mental discipline you can muster. Enduring stress while you are ill only serves to further fatigue the body, shut down the immune system, and interrupt healing.

But regardless of how tidily you might arrange your day during the *active awake* state, the *restful sleep* state must receive an even higher priority. During the *restful sleep* state, the nervous system switches to "repair" mode addressing the world *inside* the body. At rest, the body channels maximum energy to things such as immune system aggression against foreigners, immune system aggression against cancer cells,

DNA repair inside the cells, orderly cell divisions, and orderly cell deaths to keep the body's organs and structural tissue on the straight and narrow.

As an example of the role of the restful sleep state, consider that the body arrests most fevers during sleep when all hands are on the immune system deck.

Overall, each person must optimize his or her use of energy in both the awake and sleep states toward the fight with cancer. You achieve optimization by minimizing stress and by getting as much sleep as called for by your body. As you sleep, cancer cells likely die.

In Laura's case, some of the little steps we took included the following:

Excluding Laura from inclusion in the "driver pool" on interstate highway trips.

Laura did *not* attend forty of our son's all-day away baseball games, which would exhaust anyone.

Laura no longer got out of bed at the crack of dawn to let the dogs out (I actually rose to the occasion, surprising even myself).

On almost a daily basis, Laura took a hot, sea salt bath before bedtime to elevate her body temperature (as mentioned earlier) not only to relax her but also to stimulate her immune cells and to provide her body with a source of sea salt absorbed through the skin.

If Laura got worked up over something, I would gently remind her to shut the stress valve off, and so on.

We all tried to treat one another with additional kindness (a special bonus!)

When Laura returned from karate on Tuesday and Thursday nights, I always had dinner (salad and sautéed vegetables) ready for her so as not to cloud the karate exercises by creating a need or expectation for her to cook a meal, especially just as her energy reserves hit empty.

I thought I was doing well until Laura complained that I used too much olive oil in sautéing the vegetables, and she was right!

Over the course of months, calmer *active awake* and *restful sleep* states became the norm. Rather than squandering her enhanced energy levels on the outside world, we channeled these reserves where we wanted them, inside each of Laura's 100 trillion cells.

Energy! Everything suggested in this chapter is easy to do, so *do* it.

Much of my perspective on stress and survival comes from the book *Resilience* by Doctors Southwick and Charney.

OK, energy is great, but it needs oxygen, coming up next.

Chapter 14

Boosting Oxygen

*L*ast but certainly not least, *oxygen*.

Understanding Oxygen

As a basic reference point before we get started, our atmosphere currently comprises 21 percent oxygen, with the remainder nitrogen, with a little CO_2 thrown in, plus pollutants.

Evidence exists (for instance, from air trapped inside of old amber deposits) that in the past, even in the recent past, the oxygen percentage in the atmosphere may have proven higher, making it easier to breath. Now we breathe faster to gather in the equivalent volume of oxygen.

To start, let's remember that the same oxygen we bring into our bodies through our lungs corrodes almost everything it touches, and it would corrode our cells, too if that film of antioxidants did not coat them.

Good antioxidant foods in nature include things such as broccoli, kale, and sweet potatoes, but we can find many others, including berries, cherries, and lemons (or supplement concentrations of these). So far, so good; simply by eating the right foods we can arrange to bring oxygen into the cells without getting hurt in the process.

With the danger of oxygen in mind, we still need to jam endless amounts of oxygen into each cell so that the cell's mitochondria can combine oxygen with other nutrients to form ATP energy batteries.

The transportation of oxygen to the mitochondria occurs by osmosis as follows:

Oxygen concentrated in the lungs passes through lung membranes into "oxygen empty" red blood cells resulting in "oxygen filled" red blood cells, which the heart pumps forward.

At the capillary level, red blood cells come into contact with each body cell's fluid chamber. The high concentration of oxygen in the blood flows into the chamber.

From there, it enters the cell through special membrane passageways (receptors) not sensitive to the corrosive nature of oxygen.

Finally, the oxygen molecules are moved to the cell's mitochondria subchamber to oxidize food nutrients.

Conversely, once nutrients are *oxidized* (burned) and CO_2 is generated, the CO_2 gas escapes from the cell and returns to the lung to be exhaled using the same osmosis dynamics in reverse.

What can we do to help?

Oxygen Enhancement

We know that people with cancer have lower metabolized oxygen levels circulating in their bloodstreams as compared to others in the general population.

And remember, both viruses and cancer cells thrive in low-oxygen environments, so besides detoxing to elevate "oxygen friendliness," oxygen "volume"-boosting remains a must, but where to start?

Clumping — Research shows that as we age, our red blood cells start to clump while moving through the system. As an illustration, forty cells clumped together cannot grab and deliver the same amount of oxygen as forty autonomous cells because autonomous cell walls remain completely exposed at all turns allowing them to pick up a maximum amount of oxygen from the lungs and deliver that maximum to the 100 trillion cells "breathing" throughout the body.

The tiny capillaries, which bring blood down to the cellular level, are so small that red blood cells need to pass through in single file. Clumped blood never enters the capillaries; it simply circulates around the big veins and arteries never reaching the cells to deliver nutrients and oxygen.

With this as the big picture, it is safe to say that we don't like "clumping"! Before suggesting a solution to clumping, let's first try to imagine the size of the oxygen transport infrastructure in the body.

I cannot begin to estimate how many oxygen atoms we take in with every breath we breathe, so again, I will use my pretend number, "gazillions." On average, we breathe seventeen thousand times a day, and so you can imagine the elegance of the system, one that delivers an almost infinite stream of oxygen atoms to all of our 100 trillion cells on a continual basis. Any impediment to this Goliath delivery mechanism has to be bad, very bad. Each 1 percent in oxygen deficiency affects every cell in the body by 1 percent, and deeper deficiencies ultimately cause "tipping-point" enfeeblement among the cells, a recipe for viral intensity, cancer development, and tumor growth.

As I said, "We don't like clumping." It chokes off oxygen.

Laura and I use light photons to un-clump the blood as follows:

Think about photons. When the sun comes out, flowers open and turn toward that light source.

The sun's photons infuse continuous energy into every cell in the plant.

Not only does this photon bombardment cause photosynthesis (chemical stuff), it also causes THE ENTIRE PLANT TO MOVE!

We *like* **photons.** And I do mean "we," as in "us," the humans. But liking photons means more than merely enjoying a walk in the sun. Liking photons means that human cells *like* photons just the way plant cells do. Though we can't gather photons in the manner of plants (plants have leaves), our skin *does* gather photons to make things like vitamin D — *our* version of photosynthesis.

Deeper human cells, though do not enjoy exposure to the sun, but if they did, they would soak up the photon energy, supplementing the energy that the tiny mitochondria chemically produce down in the trenches.

Now, let's look at oxygen and photons in the context of "clumping" red blood cells. As a start, red blood cells contain no nucleus. Red blood cells exist merely as "temporary" quasi-cells shot out from the bone marrow to lug nutrients and oxygen around, programmed to die within thirty to sixty days. But as you age, the new red blood cells, born day-in and day-out, begin emerging in a weakened state, containing less and less energy due to the erosion of genetic data caused by overextended stem cell divisions within the bone marrow. So, they clump together in a type of old-age desperation.

Here It comes…Photon Devices

With older people, if you blast photons into the blood stream, the red clusters un-clump! (So I read.) By exposing red blood cells to a huge blast of natural photon energy, like every other cell living under the sun, the red cells know how to metabolize the incoming photon energy packets. This boost causes the tired cells to kick into gear, at least for a while, allowing the cells to unclump.

A company in Canada, called VieLight, sells such a photon delivery system. A small infrared light clip is attached into your nostril, which blasts photons for twenty-five minutes into the nasal cavity. Other than the tongue, the nasal cavity experiences the most concentrated amount of blood passing through a contained area per second. In twenty-five minutes, all the blood in the body passes through the nasal cavity, and the infrared light beam gives each red blood cell a photon boost.

Once boosted, the red cells de-clump from each other. Soon, these red cells flow through the lungs autonomously and deliver increased oxygen throughout the body — the way red blood cells do within a healthy, young, sixteen-year-old's system. By the next day, the red cells have used up their temporary photon boost and they begin clumping again, so you plug the light back into your nose, read a book, and un-clump a few billion red blood cells all over again.

The cancer cells will hate the whole experience.

By the way, photon "guns" and photon "braces" are available to "shoot" photons into, say, a sprained ankle. Injuries heal twice as fast with photon boosting. I have used this approach on four occasions with my family. That is why I knew that every cell simply LOVES photons!

Can you dig it? OK, what else?

Resveratrol

A final oxygen enhancement tactic involves opening up the blood vessels themselves. Like all parts of the body, vessel cells, too "lose altitude" as we age, and it behooves us to open them up a bit to get the blood moving freely and to deliver more oxygen faster.

How do you do this?

Well, an organic molecule called *resveratrol* does just this. Resveratrol relaxes vessels causing greater elasticity throughout vessel membranes allowing them to expand and contract with less resistance during each and every heartbeat. Blood moves fluidly, as it wants to.

Resveratrol is extracted from red grape skins and marketed in pill form. Red grape wine is known to reduce heart disease (the so called French wine effect) due to the resveratrol in the red wine, which loosens up the system reducing stress on the heart. So take resveratrol.

Now, to tie together everything said in this chapter, consider this fact as well: With her energy system tuned up to the hilt, Laura does some form of exercise daily, be it karate, jogging, or working out in the gym, which all moves lots of oxygen, lots of energy. Laura implemented this SIX DAYS A WEEK!

And speaking of blood vessel walls, don't forget about *glycation*, mentioned earlier, where sugar binds with antiaging proteins to further harden vascular channels.

Before moving beyond oxygen, please consider the following: An Alternative Cancer Theory Involving Oxygen.

Since 1931, when a Dr. Warburg won a Nobel Prize on the subject, some believe that cancer is nothing more than a normal cell whose oxygen levels have fallen to the point where the mitochondria have given up causing the cell to switch over to pure anaerobic fermentation.

Once in this state, cells cut off communication with the body, ceasing to "hear" the *apoptosis* signals to die, and so on. In this isolated state, the cells simply devour glucose and divide so long as they are fed. Toxins, smoking, poor circulation, clumping, and so on are just some of the reasons an adequate oxygen supply no longer reaches the cells.

Advocates of this theory point to another observation: the higher fermentation burn rates of aggressive cancers as compared to slow-growing cancer. High fermentation rates require a robust supply of sugar in the blood from diet.

Another complementary observation indicates that cancer cells are poisoned by oxygen once they no longer burn oxygen in a controlled setting; hence, cancer cells only experience the destructive side of oxygen.

Theories aside: Get your oxygen going...just to be sure.

Part VI

Infiltrating Cancer

Chapter 15

Send in the Trojan Horses

*I*f you follow sports, you will embrace the following: A good defense is as important as a good offense. All of this proper eating, cleanliness, immune system enhancement, oxygen boosting, and meridian energizing tactics make up your offensive attack, whereas defense means messing with your opponents—cancer cells—to drive them well out of their comfort zone.

A resourceful friend of mine advised me to have Laura ingest baking soda, as cancer hates pro-oxygen alkaline baking soda. Consuming actual baking soda seemed a very direct approach, much more aggressive than just eating alkaline-causing foods. So, I looked into it. And thus the "Trojan Horse" surfaced.

Rather than flood the blood system with backing soda that would, at best, make cancer cells somewhat uncomfortable, we found a way to trick the cancer cells into devouring large amounts of baking soda embedded in something cancer craves, a technique I referred to in the book's "Introduction" as *infiltration*. With this approach, one could "kick back" and let the cancer tumors "freak out" over their bad decision to let a wooden horse in. Two initial Trojan Horse techniques surfaced, but others followed over time.

Honey and Baking Soda

Remember how much cancer loves sugar? How it gobbles it up during PET scans? Well, the following approach infuses baking soda inside of honey and feeds the "totally" contaminated honey to the ravenous cancer cells. I like it!

The enemy "turncoat" cancer cells greedily ingest the honey and, in doing so, the intolerable amounts of backing soda hidden within stick to them like a cancer-fighting glue. The preparation for the honey-baking soda mixture follows:

- Combine half a cup of honey and half a cup of baking soda in a glass.
- Place the glass in a stovetop pan with heated water and stir for eight minutes.
- Ingest a tablespoon each day.

Hemp Oil and Frankincense Oil

This second Trojan Horse presents a similar approach: Frankincense, an *essential* oil (must be ingested), confuses cancer cells over whether to divide or not as the frankincense somehow inhibits the division trigger. To get the "traitorous" cancer cells to ingest the frankincense, the frankincense is mixed into CBD hemp oil by a Colorado firm called Bluebird.

Note: By "essential," medical people mean that the body cannot make the compound in question internally, and hence, if you want the compound, it is "essential" to ingest it from outside the body.

CBD oil is gleaned from hemp plants, which we once used to make rope. CBD molecules happen to have receptors that match up with cancer cell receptors, so that by ingesting hemp oil, you effectively coat the cancer tumor with hemp gook, which itself, like an antibody, attracts immune cells.

By mixing in some frankincense with the hemp oil, you have delivered a double blow to the tumor. The CBD oil first serves as an antibody beacon to lure immune cells, and second, through osmosis, the tumor absorbs the unwanted frankincense right into its gut.

It's a two-for-one deal! Screw 'em!

Intravenous Vitamin C Considered

Some alternative-therapy practitioners, including the aforementioned Mexican doctor, advocate intravenous injection of mega-doses of vitamin C. The direct injection of the vitamin prevents the digestive tract from compromising the C molecule. Proponents claim that the body converts concentrated C into substances that affect the anaerobic mechanism these rogue cells depend upon.

The derived compound contains H_2O_2 (hydrogen peroxide), which, in turn, floods cancer cells with unwanted oxygen. Because you need to have an IV installed, we did not look further into this therapy but hope that science can get closer to it as it seems a plausible construct.

Other advocates suggest bypassing the mega C step and simply ingesting low dosages of hydrogen peroxide in distilled water. We also passed on this for now as I feared using an incorrect dosage.

OK, everything described so far took place over the first ninety days of the plan. There was more to come.

Part VII

Grit and Grace

Chapter 16

Month 3— Breakthrough

The Ninety-Day Photograph

Almost ninety days passed since we learned of the cancer. Time for another trip to New York City to remeasure Laura's tumors using the 3D sonogram; time to determine if anything we were doing or thinking works.

It started good and ended, shall we say...well, you'll see...We set our meeting with the doctor for 2:30 p.m. as inspired planning allowed time for lunch in Manhattan. So we enjoyed lunch with Toni and Vinnie, our best New York City friends ever. At lunch, spirits remained high based simply upon Laura's "look" and energy, and simply at our pleasure in sitting with people of our inner circle especially at lunch on Manhattan's Columbus Circle. We left the restaurant confident never losing our core conviction that things were working; yet, as we walked the hot, midtown New York City streets on the way to the doctor's office, each New York City block became heavier and hotter!

The doctor's office felt extremely warm since we had just crossed midtown in the blazing sun, so we "sweated," waiting our turn to receive the verdict. Finally, the receptionist gives us the sign and takes us to one of the examination rooms. The good Doctor (and I *mean* it) walks in and instantly engages us as if we had just seen each other earlier that day.

Today, he is all business, as he, too wants to see what has transpired across recent time. He spots the titanium markers sitting inside of the right breast and looks for the tumors. We follow the analysis on the screen monitor.

"The smaller one is no longer visible," the Doctor pronounces calmly. A half-a-minute later, he proclaims, "The bigger tumor has shrunken by half."

That's it? After all of those months, days, and hours, it took but a mere minute or two to determine that, "we were good"? Witnessing the evidence on the video screens with my own two eyes, I next remember paying the $800 bill and leaving. During it all, Laura and I show no sign of joy whatsoever. We had steeled ourselves not to react to news, good *or* bad.

Walking up the street, Laura asks, "Shouldn't we be happy?"

I answer, "We are."

Our next 3-D sonogram appointment would take place 150 days out.

Next Steps and Daily Life

Do you remember I told you how I found my first wife chain-smoking cigarettes saying that her fight days were over? Well, the self-healing plan is a long-range strategy, and the plan absolutely warrants flexibility to cultivate stamina and your ability to stick with it. And so, driving out of Manhattan to finally celebrate, I pull the car over and get Laura a slice of pizza. But after that, it was "back to basics" plan-wise, yet not at the intensity maintained during the first ninety days. Leading up to the 3-D ultrasound checkup, Laura, over a stretch of twenty-one days, went "super-extreme" in consuming a zero-sugar-and-fat diet while eating only alkaline vegetables for a truly inspiring run of discipline. As a result, the good news regarding tumor shrinkage meant this: *Laura's whole body had taken up the offensive – and it was winning.*

So, we should keep it up, right?

Yes, but you run the 100-yard dash differently than the New York City marathon. So, use the momentum of the good results as the fuel source for a long run, right? Let's not burn up willpower by forcing endless 100-yard sprints.

The first ninety days proved special in other ways as well. For one, they addressed the excess triglycerides and toxins sitting inside Laura's 100 trillion cells and had "shown them the door" with conviction. Laura, now at her young woman's weight, had met these essential milestones.

On day 90, Laura's nourishment was solely supplied by what she ate *that day* and not by long-forgotten substances buried inside her body for decades. The flow of glucose and keytones through her body was even and moderated to the level needed by healthy cells. This meant that we could alter the plan to some degree, something that the holistic doctor had also recommended.

Laura started by eating fish and chicken every other day while still depriving the ever-shrinking cancer colonies. Watching Laura go off to karate each day, I felt better that we had reintroduced some low-fat, semi-alkaline sources of protein. For the next 150 days, Laura continued to consume fish or chicken every other day.

Still, there were no gushing sugar spikes coming in to relieve the cancer (though later I would uncover more insight into subtle sugar spikes and diabetic conditions, described at the end of the book).

And so, day by day, we plug on with imperfect confidence. Time would tell.

Chapter 17

Month 8—Almost There

The Plan

At the end of October, the schedule called for us to return to New York City to have a third 3-D sonogram image compiled of her large tumor (you'll recall that the small tumor had already disappeared by the time of the second sonogram five months earlier). We felt pretty confident that the results would prove good as Laura had stuck to the already-effective self-healing plan all along. But more so, throughout this second four-month tenure with her body clear of toxins and triglyceride reserves and her immune system empowered, she had truly *deprived* and persistently *infiltrated* the cancer.

By September, seven months in, Laura had settled into her new weight, her ideal 113 pounds—the same as in her twenties. She looked and felt great, with her cells living in a nontoxic environment, with plenty of oxygen, vigorous immune responses, reduced microbe activity, passive cancer remnants, and no sugar, caffeine, or alcohol-like stimulants and a steady flow of alkaline-tilting nutrients. Laura's system hummed.

And so, like a closing pitcher in Major League Baseball, it came time to *really* pour it on. By this I mean bringing her life energy up to a higher plane by introducing the double helix water and the CoQ10 supplements (already described) to deliver the "final blows" to end the war, at least for now. The double helix water would heighten electrical energy inside every cell in the body, spurring each cell's mitochondria to gear up as the CoQ10 fed the mitochondria the enzyme they needed to work at this elevated level.

We set another goal for October "to live a little," to get fresh psychological momentum transitioning into the upcoming Living Wisely phase of the plan (though this would backfire should the late October test bring bad news). I called this "The October Offensive." But before launching the troops, so to speak, first we took stock in where we stood.

The Kinseologist

The kinseologist found no remaining issues in Laura's energy-balancing status.

The Biological Dentist

The biological dentist retested Laura for toxins (pesticides, heavy metals, fungi, preservatives, tooth and gut microbe excretions, etc.) and found no remaining levels. As we never removed her root canal tooth, he captured an electronic image of possible microbe toxins emanating from the tooth and made a special water vial from this image for Laura to take in October.

The Naturopath Doctor

Doctor Vincent took a blood test to check Laura's levels. Almost every category had become optimal. For example, Laura's triglycerides now ran just 43 rather than 130. Her vitamin levels placed well within range, and her thyroid numbers were good though her white blood count was slightly elevated.

A Special Blood Test

Months earlier, during one of my research nights, I stumbled upon the serum TK blood test (to my knowledge, no longer available) that tests for the degree of cell division in the body. As some cells die and others divide (the programmed apoptosis and mitosis routines previously described), the process leaves a certain by-product serum behind in the bloodstream. If cancer is on the rise with millions of cells abnormally dividing, this serum level rises at a measurable rate.

I purchased two test packages online. We would get a baseline test of Laura's serum level now, in October of 2014, using the first test pack to benchmark cell division as it currently stood, and then we planned to measure activity later on, say, in six months' time, using the second test pack. After killing off the visible cancer, we would need a "trust and verify" scheme, and this was to be part of it (a second, similar test surfaced later as well).

The results of the serum TK test indicated that cancer activity still existed somewhere in Laura's system. But we now had a specific serum level to use going forward to gauge positive or negative cell division momentum.

Double Helix Water, Revisited

With all of these preparations in hand, I called the double helix water people again. I mentioned earlier that I had contacted their California office to discuss the concept and the history of this hard-to-imagine find. Since that initial call, I had read the book published by Doctors Gann and Lo, the two scientists behind it all. I called Jon, the fellow I had previously spoken to. I again found him communicative, able to discuss matters at any level — theoretical, testing, plan, and so on.

I asked about the relative concentration of double helix water molecules in regular water as compared to the vials of water they would send me.

Each vial would contain one million more double helix molecules than tap or seawater. These would be distributed throughout the body in a pro rata manner across 100 trillion cells (remember, the body is 70 percent water). Because of the number of cells (100 trillion), the plan for breast cancer meant ingesting seven vials of double helix water each day. This would raise the standing electrical charge in each cell to an optimal level, double the charge a typical older person carries due to a dwindling "power supply." The elevated charge, spread and pulsated via the meridian system, would push every cell to operate at its eighteen-year-old potential. The mitochondria would spin for all they were worth, and the Q10would provide the mitochondria sufficient fuel to operate comfortably at this aggressive pace. Presumably, cells would no longer tolerate viruses, and immune cells would "take no prisoners" in their pursuit of foreign (antigen) invaders.

I ordered a whole bunch of vials, and we purchased some CoQ10 from a health food store.

Literature describes CoQ10 as a *coenzyme*. This bothered me, as the "co" designation meant that a partner enzyme was needed but none was ever mentioned. In 2018, new literature surfaced describing the missing link, an organic molecule called QPP. Together, CoQ10 and QPP not only provide the mitochondria with fuel, but QPP represents the most powerful antioxidant known, a "reducing agent" vastly more potent than vitamin C. QPP is listed in the "Appendix."

An American Indian Remedy

For centuries, a famous tea consisting of forest matter used by American Indians from the Toronto area earned a reputation for thwarting cancer. I do not know why so many believe it works, but so many sources had mentioned this tea over the past months that I decided to throw it into the mix now, in October 2014, for good measure. We bought some at a health food store and Laura drank it until we ran out.

Let's Roll

OK, our October plan is in place, what else? Oh yeah… "Live a little."

Laura wears her New York Giants Fan heart on her sleeve with Eli Manning the entire New York Giant franchise in her eyes. For years, I have watched Laura scream bloody murder at Eli on national television should he commit the slightest miscue. Thankfully, the attack does not fall solely upon Eli. For instance, Laura's scathing criticism buried Eli's big brother Peyton throughout the 2014 Super Bowl, a worse attack from Laura than Peyton experienced from that West Coast team, whoever *they* were (the Seahawks, of course).

Eli, though, does gain relief from criticism whenever Laura attacks the refs, such as when the opposition tackled Eli in the end zone gaining two points for the deed *and* possession of the ball (it's called a "safety"). Laura followed this decision against the Giants with accusations of cash exchanges and referee corruption taking place right on national TV, with Laura, of course, the only person in America to see through it all.

Then there was the play where an opposition wide receiver circled back and executed the old Statue of Liberty "handoff" from his own quarterback advancing twenty yards. Laura went ballistic, screaming, "Where the hell are the refs, doesn't anyone else see this? They just stole their own ball!"

My favorite game: The time Eli threw a bunch of interceptions against Green Bay. From several rooms away, I heard her screaming, "Eli, you know what you are? You're (expletive deleted)."

I came running in to learn the cause of the commotion and Laura blurted out, "Eli keeps throwing the ball to the guys in the green outfits."

Well, you get the point, "Giants or death," though I prefer, "Live free or die."

On Saturday night, October 6th, at 11 p.m., the dam broke, and I decided to buy good seats on Stubhub for Laura, me, and our son, Joseph, for the very next day's game, Sunday, October 7th, against the Atlanta Falcons. The game started at 1 p.m. at MetLife Stadium in Rutherford, New Jersey. It meant six hours of round-trip driving time, which violated the "no stress" plan, but so what! Laura did not plan on eating those stadium hot dogs, washing them down with the $12 beers, so we left early, went to a local store, and bought her special grub to bring into the stadium.

Of course, there were two automobile accidents on the George Washington Bridge, one on the upper level and one on the lower. We sat in the snarled traffic and Laura's blood began to boil. She agreed to calm down. No need to produce cortisol over a slight delay in the plan.

It was Laura's first time in the stands at an NFL game. The sun glowed brightly producing a perfect 65-degree day, and the Giants had just scored as we entered the stadium, late by twenty minutes. Atlanta scored as we found our seats. Eli next threw a few bad passes, and Atlanta scored twice more. Laura sat devastated going into halftime. In the second half, Eli finally found his game, pounding away, finding Cruz and Beckham. Laura had her chance to scream in unison with the thousands of Giants fans and exchange multiple high-fives, and we departed with a 30 to 20 Giant comeback victory notched on her belt.

Thank you, Eli, *thank* you.

Crossing back over the George Washington Bridge, we passed Columbia Presbyterian Hospital, and I recalled that troubling episode months earlier and reflected upon how far Laura had come in a relatively small number of months with her *own* second-half comeback.

The Third 3-D Sonogram

A few weeks later, we were back in New York to see Doctor Bard and get a third 3-D sonogram measurement of the remaining tumor. The results were good as the tumor had flattened out. It was the same length, but it had lost most of its depth and width.

On this visit, Doctor Bard prescribed his own supplements, a strong concoction of primrose-based antioxidants, some CoQ10, and something to temper the dense breast tissue situation, which he explained resulted in four times the occurrence of breast cancer (more on dense breast tissue later).

We left in good spirits.

Chapter 18

Month 12—No Tumors

It's Been a Year

Finally, in February of 2015, Laura's one-year check-up date arrived.

The last tumor measurement had taken place in October 2014, four months before. Back then, no sign of the smaller tumor appeared, but the shrunken, larger tumor remained visible. Now, after another 120 days, we would find out if the gods continued to smile upon us.

Laura stayed on track during those 120 days…well, sort of. First during Thanksgiving, and then during Christmas and New Year's, she had indulged in various food liberties on multiple occasions. Overall, though, Laura followed 80 percent of the plan. She took her supplements, continued her exercise, and her food consumption never included sugar, carbohydrates, or acidic red meat. Yes, a glass of red wine had become standard fare with dinner with chicken and fish almost daily.

Still, Laura worried that she had let up on the gas pedal. I reminded her that a) she still followed the plan at the 80 percent level, and b) that all of the detoxification benefits accrued during the first six months of the plan remained in place. Her acidic toxins were gone. But she noticed that from a weight of 113 pounds for almost a year, on January 10 the scale suddenly read 118. (Quietly, I gulped—wrong direction!)

The drive into Manhattan from our Connecticut residence typically takes two-and-a-half hours, but anything can happen once you get near the city. To avoid unknown delays, we decided to drive halfway to the city, stopping in Brewster, New York, to park the car and take the Metro North commuter train into Grand Central Terminal on 42nd Street.

Arriving in the city at 11:45 a.m., we head through the frigid streets making our way to 44th Street and a favorite New York destination, the Greek seafood restaurant Kellari Taverna. While enjoying all of the restaurant's great energy and food, I ask Laura if she feels nervous about her doctor's appointment.

Her answer: "There's nothing that can be done now, so why worry?"

We had grown measured and even stoic over the course of the year.

The doctor, happy to see us, appears generally optimistic, although before getting started he cautions: "These things can get better, but they can slip backward, too. Let's take a look..."

Laura goes off with a physician's assistant for a mammogram. Next, we sit in the waiting room until we are asked to step into the doctor's office.

"Well, I have good news. The mammogram does not show any tumors. The two titanium markers are visible, but no sign of tumors. Let's go into the examination room and try the sonogram."

The doctor examines both breasts and the lymph nodes in each armpit, saying that all of the nodes are clear. Then he goes back to the right breast.

"I still see something where the large tumor was… it may be the last remnant of the tumor, or it may be scar tissue, but at least we have a picture of it for future reference. I can also tell you that the breast density found on previous visits has been reduced." Looking us in the eye, he notes: "Dense breast tissue is a marker for development of new occurrences, so the improvement is very encouraging."

Please recall that four months ago, Dr. Bard had prescribed his own brand of antioxidants and vascular support supplements designed to address both antioxidant goals and the breast density issue. Recall that a key objective is to eliminate chronic inflammation caused by oxidative stress as inflammation encourages cancer cell divisions. Looks like Doctor Bard's "patented" supplements worked.

And, with a smile, he says: "You two should go home and not worry about this for six months. Come back in the summer and we'll take another look."

Privately, "the Irish" side of me was going to worry "a wee bit" longer!

Then he turned to me and asks: "What about you? I see you haven't come in for a prostate exam. You should be tested every six months." (The 3-D sonogram system is used for prostate examinations as well). I agree to sign up for an exam when we return in the summer.

We hop a cab to Grand Central Station and head home. While on the train, I send a text out to our four children telling them the good news.

Now What?

Driving home from the Brewster train station, Laura brought the subject up, saying, "The doctor seemed a little cryptic."

I weighed in, "He reported as clearly as possible. The mammogram showed no tumors and we'd look at the tumor sites again in six months' time to check the residue tissue."

"Then can I cut back on taking some of these pills?" she mused.

"I don't know," I replied. "Everything you take has a clear purpose. Let's just get through this week and we can regroup next week."

By "getting through this week," I referred to my own immediate travel plans and Laura's second-tier black belt test coming up in a few days' time. The next day, I take off on a three-day side trip to New Orleans with my oldest daughter Codyann; she is doing research for her undergraduate thesis and I am tagging along. I wished that Laura could make the Louisiana trip as well, but she needed to stay home to train and rest to prepare for her second-degree black belt test that coming Sunday.

I had mixed feelings about the black belt event only because it is a big deal physically. You fight ten opponents for one minute each with the karate master demanding, "I want to see you fight!" In "plan-think," this means huge amounts of cortisol created by the body in an ultimate "fight or flight" scenario. And I worried not just about those ten minutes of constant battle; leading up to fight day, Laura would hone her fighting chops as well as her cardiovascular stamina with daily prep sessions. To me, this meant even more cortisol, more lactic acid, and more inflammation.

But still, I knew I had a fighter on my hands, and fighting is what a fighter does.

As I leave for Louisiana, Laura agrees to take the hot baths each night so that her body can switch off the combat hormones and induce the sleep and rest hormones. We touch base each day.

Black Belts

When I return from Louisiana on Saturday evening, Laura appears tired but ready for her Sunday promotion test the next morning. At the "dojo" (Japanese karate centers are called *dojos*), I recognize many senior black belt veterans from previous years who had traveled from different locations across America to attend, with many 5th-degree black belt masters in attendance as well, both male and female. That day, Laura would fight ten of them. Other black belts up for promotion fight before her, and one fellow gets hurt tearing his ACL. It is tough, grim business, and I cringe watching each punch or kick that is landed.

Then comes Laura's good friend Audrey's turn. One by one, the international master calls ten challengers up, and Audrey starts to hammer away. With her first opponent,

Audrey's right hand gets cut. Next, during her spar with the second challenger, her left knuckle is cut. As Audrey lands punches, blood stains the white smocks (called *ghis* in Japanese) of each opponent. After five challengers, a woman runs out to place bandages on Audrey's hands, but Kaicho, the master, calls her off as this would allow Audrey to catch her breath.

"It doesn't matter. Fight!"

Finally, it ends. I turn to Audrey's husband and joke, "Well, she bloodied every one of them."

His response: "Too bad it's her blood."

Laura stands up, wanting to fight next.

Laura does not hold back. High kicks and punching flourishes continued through the first four fights, until she takes a bad kick to her left leg and staggers. She gets kicked there again by the next fighter, and the master yells to keep fighters from going after that leg while still demanding that the fight continues with full force. A veteran, Laura keeps her energy source as aerobic, pacing herself, relaxing even while in combat to keep her breathing at its optimum level. But by fighter number eight, her aerobic stamina wanes. Her willpower triggers the painful anaerobic creation of energy lasting until the finish. It goes on and on and finally it ends. Almost!

The master tells Laura to do twenty-five knuckle push-ups. At twenty-five, the master calls for ten more, then ten more, and then ten more.

Standing up, Laura next has to kick ten tennis balls hanging from the ceiling above her head. If she misses one, the count starts over. She gets five and misses number six. At some point she reaches ten, five kicked with her right leg and five with her injured left leg.

Next, the master gives Laura a broomstick, which she holds with both hands. While holding it, she must jump over the broomstick so that it ends up behind her and then jump back to bring the broomstick forward again. She must complete this task ten times while the *dojo* counts in Japanese. If she stumbles, the count begins anew. Laura stumbles more than once, until her vast power of the mind takes over, and she cleanly jumps back-and-forth ten times.

"Enough!" the master proclaims.

The room applauds as Laura, drenched in perspiration, sits down next to Audrey.

Chapter 19

Digging Deeper

The Next Phase Is Upon Us

"Next week" comes quickly; time to regroup and talk about the plan going forward.

Laura and I chat first about food. Laura says she does not want to change her diet. For instance, she now loves kale and beets and finds red meat revolting. When we visit a steakhouse, Laura will flip directly to the chicken and fish options on the menu.

Yes, Laura takes a lot of supplements—well-targeted supplements—and if you crush all of the pills, it only comes to a small pile of dust ingested along with the three-to-four quarts of food and liquid she consumes each day. Regardless of these "reasonable" proportions, Laura's tolerance for taking pills is sinking fast. But rather than expecting her to reduce her supplements, I had secretly uncovered additional supplements that I itched to pitch to her.

Enzymes

For example, we could now consider the topic of enzymes. As I mentioned earlier, I held off on this topic throughout the whole year of the plan other than adding CoQ10, which, technically, constitutes a coenzyme that is used by the mitochondria to convert incoming nutrients into energy. In general, *enzymes* are internally created chemicals made by the body that cause other chemical reactions to take place. Enzymes are *catalysts*, but they need other players such as coenzymes to work their magic.

Enzymes operate down in the chemical trenches of your bodily fluids causing *chemical by-products*; they are not to be confused with *hormones*, chemical triggers operating at a higher level directing *cellular behavior*.

The body creates and deploys thousands of enzymes to cause a host of chemical-transposing results such as breaking down food in the intestines. You might consider taking digestive enzymes, for example, as a supplement.

First an aside: For the purposes of fighting cancer, some advocate that certain enzyme supplements can "spur on" the immune system and that other enzymes can "corrode" the walls of cancer cells. I could find nothing to substantiate these claims, so I passed on these, but my ears remain open.

Another example: When you get hurt, inflammation (think "sticky goo") takes place, causing pain so that the body stays quiet while healing steps take place. Enzymes eventually move in to corrode the inflammation to flush it out of the system, relieving pain. OK, so different centers of the body create thousands of enzyme components addressing thousands of biological objectives.

Finally, I find one enzyme that focuses on reducing breast fibrosis by eliminating scar tissue as follows.

Scar Tissue and Breast Density

I don't know how many times I heard and read that women with dense breast tissue are four times as likely to get breast cancer than woman without dense breast tissue. Yet no one, and no writing I could find, suggested a) why dense breast tissue (*fibrosis*) occurred in the first place, or b) why dense tissue would lead to four times the occurrence of breast cancer for these women.

Now that Laura and I had destroyed the tumors, I pondered this four-times-as-likely topic, figuring that if not confronted, any propensity for fresh cancer occurrences would be unchecked allowing cancer to repropagate.

So I asked myself: "What the heck do they mean by 'dense breast tissue,' and why could this condition lead to disease?" Thankfully, Susan G Komen on her breast cancer website explains the following:

"*Breast density* is not a measure of how the breasts feel, but rather how the breasts look on a mammogram. *High-breast density* means there is a greater amount of breast connective tissue (fibrosis) as compared to fat. *Low-breast density* means there is a greater amount of fat as compared to breast and connective tissue."

OK, get ready to contemplate the following idea. If correct, breast cancer sufferers and all aging persons will sing "halleluiah"!

What is scar tissue?

Have you ever thought of this?

Again, what is scar tissue? You have heard about it all of your life!

First, *scar tissue* is not alive. It is a string of proteins that certain guardian cells create whenever the body suffers damage. Ejected protein strings from the guardians bind damaged tissue together until it heals. So, *scar tissue* is a bunch of chemical strings that envelope damaged cells and leftover stocks of inflammation gook. All of this stuff is DEAD!

Wise GEEK explained scarring as follows:

"Internal scar tissue can be formed by various causes including repetitive usage. The healing process will begin by forming fibrosis tissue around the injury, effectively forming a web that protects it from further harm.

"During this stage, the injured cells turn into *adhesions*, which are basically dead cells. The fibrosis tissue, along with a body chemical known as *collagen*, then begins working to repair the damaged area with new cells. As the area heals, the adhesions that were present will develop into permanent scar tissue."

Fundamentally, we should not refer to it as scar "tissue" as tissue implies living cells fed by blood and lymph networks. Scars are simply dead organic masses that often stay with you until you die. Personally, I have all kinds of scar tissue buried in my body due to injury and age, so I get it. And it hurts!

So I looked into both "stringy scar tissue" and the "inflammatory goo" which the body's neutrophil immune cells mindlessly park around traumatized tissues. What I found: The body, apparently, makes enzymes that rid these necessary evils once they have done their job. Two interesting enzymes called wobenzyme-N and seffaflazyme surfaced. They apparently corrode inflammatory goo and scar tissue itself. Research in the 1990s by a Doctor Lee isolated these enzymes.

We apparently create anti-inflammatory and anti-scarring enzymes in large quantities only up until the age of twenty-seven; and perhaps that explains why younger people can come back from injury much faster and better than older people. The construct of these "injury mop-up" enzymes is as follows:

Both young and old bodies create scar "tissue" to mend injured tissue. With younger bodies, scarring represents a temporary step toward full rehabilitation of the damaged tissue. After the string-like scar protein has done its job—holding the damaged area together—the scar-busting enzymes come in and corrode the scar fibers away so that primary tissue can fill in where scar matter once resided.

Because older people (past age twenty-seven) have reduced supplies of these enzymes, they tend to accumulate scar proteins as the years go by, never purging them, and they learn to live with the chronic inflammation that scarring, a foreign substance, evokes.

The Big Idea (Finally)

My proposition: Fibrosis of the breast is nothing more than scar fibers resulting from the monthly wear and tear of the menstrual cycle. As breast cells divide and die each month, bits of fibrosis result building up over decades. The fibrosis scar and inflammation goo clogs everything up, making the breast tissue "dense." As a result of the clutter, some women have reduced blood and lymph support to combat viruses. Budding cancer colonies incubate among the good fat cells suffocating within the breast. So, if breast density claims nothing more than string-like, scarred fibers and inflammatory goo, would the wobenzyme-N and seffaflazyme enzymes help ameliorate the "density" condition?

The idea for adding wobenzyme-N and seffalazyme as supplements is threefold:

First, they will reverse some of the aging effects of scar tissue throughout the body caused by a lifetime of traumatic *skeletal* injuries.

Second, *micro-scar* tissue and chronic inflammatory deposits accumulated due to wear and tear in the organs can also be reduced systemically (body-wide), providing greater vascular support to these workhorse organs.

Third, in the case of dense-breast conditions, the enzyme might corrode some of the fibrosis and inflammatory deposits, restoring vascular support—providing nutrients, oxygen, and immune cells—that will keep breast cells healthier going forward.

This might be too good to be true, but if nature has created a complex enzyme to perfectly address scar tissue and inflammation, then I would trust this natural compound.

Note: I personally tried wobenzyme first as a test case. A week into it, I drove one college daughter three hours to school on a Saturday and a second daughter six hours to school the next day, Sunday. Pulling up to the driveway at the end of the Sunday marathon, I feared stepping out of the car. In recent years, car time meant pain time. Yet, I stood up with minimal stiffness.

A week later, I realized that I was sleeping on both sides, though previously, due to rotator cuff shoulder injuries, I could last but fifteen minutes on a side without triggering massive shoulder pain.

If my chronic inflammation could be reduced by enzymes, then why not breast density (and the inflammation deposits of Crone's disease as well)?

Due to this manifest result within my own body, Laura added six weeks of the more aggressive seffaflazyme to the plan at the start of the "trust and verify" phase, and then added the milder wobenzyme-N.

Blood Tests

In anticipation of the Doctor Bard visit to visually reexamine the tumor sites via his 3-D sonogram, in parallel, I organized two blood tests to uncover any chemical markers indicating ongoing cancer activity within Laura's body: 1) another serum TK test (described earlier) to measure Laura's current degree of internal cell division, and 2) a new test, called ONCOBLOT, that looks for unique protein by-products in the bloodstream each made by a specific cancer cell type.

I ordered the serum TK test kit online and had blood drawn locally and sent it off to the lab.

ONCOBLOT was new, a test made available just recently based upon breakthrough research that isolated certain unique proteins excreted by twenty-six different cancer cell types. These "marker" proteins, if found floating around in your bloodstream, indicate cancer activity — breast, lung, colon, and so on — even if tumors are not yet visible. Here is a blog description of ONCOBLOT by a Doctor Chris Foley:

"The best imaging detects cancer only after it has grown to ~ 1 billion cells or more, yet this test can detect cancer that is only 2 million cells large—perhaps months or years before you could see it on a mammogram, colonoscopy, or with a PSA blood test. Maybe there are very less invasive, toxic, or expensive ways to eradicate it long before it becomes a serious illness. "Microscopic cancer" may become a new entity, detected, then eradicated long before a conventional test or worse, symptoms, indicate its presence. Also, if one has had cancer in the past and is being subjected to ongoing scans and tests to detect evidence of recurrence, this could greatly improve the accuracy and reduce radiation exposure."

Laura's long-time endocrinologist, Doctor Raffaele in New York, who treated her for thyroid issues, told me about this cutting-edge blood test. After understanding the achievements of ONCOBLOT lab's capabilities, Laura and I went to Doctor Raffaele's New York City office, and we both had blood drawn and sent away to the ONCOBLOT lab for evaluation (to see if any of the cancer-specific proteins they had in their database matched up with proteins found in our blood samples). Our results are discussed in the next chapter.

Chapter 20

Not So Fast

*O*K, here comes yet another trip into New York City. This time, we went the night before, stayed at the Crown Plaza hotel right in the heart of Times Square, had dinner, and went to a comedy club. Here is what transpired the next day:

Our first doctor's appointment began at 9:30 a.m. with Doctor Raffaele, the endocrinologist just mentioned, who monitors Laura's biochemical health. This would be followed at 1:30 p.m. by a Doctor Bard appointment to scan for visible signs of cancer using his fancy 3-D sonogram and Doppler systems.

Blood Markers

Three weeks before on our last New York trip, Doctor Raffaele had drawn blood from both Laura and me and sent the vials to OCONOBLOT to test for traces of cancer. OCONOBLOT, if you recall, only as of 2014, identifies

---

cancer-specific proteins in your blood serum with each cancer type releasing its own special protein.

So far, OCONOBLOT has identified twenty-six unique cancer proteins. According to OCONOBLOT, 2 million cancer cells need to be active to put out enough measurable protein for this test. In comparison, visible tumors house from 500 million cells to hundreds of billions, so this cutting-edge blood test identifies problems very early on, perhaps years in advance of detecting cancer by mammograms, MRIs, PET scans, and so on. Doctor Raffaelle had also sent other blood samples to his regular lab to look into Laura's blood, hormone, and vitamin levels.

My ONCOBLOT test came back giving me a clean bill of health; no sign of any of the twenty-six cancers lurking in my body. As we expected, Laura's test indicated that her breast cancer was still active. All of her other numbers across the other blood tests were excellent. Doctor Raffaele, Laura, and I mused what to do with this information. If everyone over fifty took the ONCOBLOT test, many hidden cases of cancer would suddenly show panicking many people possibly over nothing. For example, if you had colon cancer proteins in the blood, would that justify undergoing chemotherapy that affects your entire body just to thwart a yet invisible cancer colony? This level of protein testing certainly opens the door to new treatment dilemmas and options. Maybe self-healing will be looked at as one of them.

In Laura's case, knowing that her body had just killed billions of breast cancer cells, the findings meant one thing: *Give her immune system more time to ferret out the remaining cells and reduce their numbers to a chemically undetectable level.* I propose that anyone who takes the OCONOBLOT test and discovers lurking cancer do the same. Use self-healing plans to reverse the cancer colony's progress long before it can even be seen.

We decided to schedule another ONCOBLOT test six months out.

OK, time for lunch. We had two hours to kill before our appointment with Doctor Bard. We walk three blocks to Nello, a top Italian restaurant on Madison Avenue. Laura and I both order salad and Dover sole with a bottle of Rose-de-Provence to boot. Lunch was delightful. Unlike a year before where we had shared many a quiet moment, we were quite chatty this time.

From Nello, another three blocks farther east is Doctor Bard's office. While sitting in his waiting room, he surfaces momentarily, and I mention that I have new information. In the examination room, Doctor Bard goes right to work setting up for three different scans of Laura's chest cavity and lymph nodes, and he asks me to convey the new information. I tell him about the two blood tests:

Red Drop—which indicates excess or runaway cell division in the body by testing your TK serum levels. Cell division in both normal and cancerous cells generates TK; too much TK means more cell division (cancer) than normal.

I told him that we had done a few of these Red Drop tests, that Laura's TK numbers were still slightly out of normal range but had improved drastically over the course of the year as her tumors shrank. This was our *macro* way of gauging Laura's cancer momentum.

OCONOBLOT—which tests for specific proteins released by each cancer type, was our *micro* way of gauging Laura's cancer presence. This new test, just available recently, indicated low-level breast cancer activity somewhere in Laura's body (tissue or lymph glands).

This got the good doctor going. He concentrated deeply, running his scans, looking for anything evil, finally giving up, and saying that both breasts and all of the lymph nodes looked completely normal. The inert tissue where the large tumor once resided was still there, but identical in condition to where it stood six months before: that is, it was scar tissue with no vascular interaction.

I handed him a piece of paper with "Red Drop – macro" and "OCONOBLOT – micro" written on it. He went into his office, we to the waiting room. Minutes went by, and Laura asked what was going on. I said that undoubtedly Doctor Bard was online looking up the tests. Sure enough when we were brought into his office, he had already deciphered the claims of both tests. He did not exactly say that they were bogus offerings but warned that in medicine there are hundreds of breakthrough claims appearing as the next big thing only to collapse a year out.

I mentioned that with twenty-six cancer tests to perform, OCONOBLOT found nothing in me and the correct protein out of twenty-six for Laura. And that over the past year, Laura's Red Drop TK serum numbers dropped commensurate with her tumor shrinkage – pretty good evidence that both are viable testing options.

As Doctor Bard has a busy travel schedule attending many medical conventions and presenting his advanced diagnostic tools, he said he would dig deeper into these tests with his colleagues. But assuming they are valid, he held that Laura's known progress was what counted, and with self-healing tools in place, we should not consider invasive tactics. We made an appointment for six months out.

So what's next? Next was a trip to Georgia and a week of travel to attend the baseball competitions for our son's Connecticut team. A year before, Laura did not go on this stressful and fatiguing trip as part of the "no stress" principle, but there was no stopping her this time around. The next day, we arrived in Atlanta where it was 101 degrees.

Over the next days, the topic came up as what to do about squeezing the remaining cancer out. Laura's take was to reinstate the *infiltration* leg of the plan. It had been months since she had consumed the honey and baking soda concoction and ingested the CBD oil and frankincense supplement; the CBD bottle had been dropped and was broken and we had not even reordered one.

I said fine, we'll get those going, but I found a third infiltration option, *saffron,* from an article in *Life Extension Magazine.* Saffron, like frankincense, slows cancer down and has three organic molecules that blunt cancer's propensity to divide and multiply. A week later the new supplements arrive, and infiltration takes the lead role going forward. Now we wait. Months later in December of 2015, we did three blood tests:

White Blood Cell Nutritional Measurements – to ensure Laura's mineral and vitamin levels were in range.

Red Drop's TK Serum Test – to gauge Laura's cell division level as measured against the general population.

OCONOBLOT – To detect the microscopic presence of cancer.

We discuss the test results and what we did in response to them in our next, final chapter.

Chapter 21

Digging Even Deeper

*I*t is December of 2015, nineteen months since Laura was diagnosed with breast cancer from that original mammogram. The nutrient report comes in looking good, but the Red Drop and OCONOBLOT reports give us pause. Laura's Red Drop number had not changed from what it had been six months before. The Red Drop ranges are as follows:

20 or Less	—	Normal range of TK activity
21-40	—	Moderate TK activity
41-80	—	Precancerous levels of TK activity
81-120	—	Risk of developing cancer
121 and Over	—	Active cancer range

Laura had a 37, the "Moderate Level," whatever that means. I call Red Drop, and their view is that a steady 37 is nothing to fret about considering the higher TK levels found when people carry visible cancer, and especially since Laura had been twice that level at some point.

Optimism is good, I guess, but I also had the ONCOBLOT report in hand saying that traces of breast cancer were still kicking. And so, though I accepted the encouragement the people at Red Drop offered, I knew that a multiyear push was still needed to squash the remaining cancer strongholds. But still, after all that Laura and I had done over the past nineteen months to get this far, I was beside myself as to where the final push would come from. As it happened, at this very juncture of befuddlement, Laura's father and my father-in-law, Phil, was struggling with diabetes. He was slim and yet still was in trouble. I decided to look into this for Phil's sake, and I soon stumbled onto an insight that might explain how to resolve the last of Laura's cancer cell holdouts.

A Connection between Diabetes and Cancer

Earlier in the book, I described a sugar absorption test Laura underwent where a Russian doctor determined that after a meal, Laura's blood sugar levels remained high for too long. Since then, Laura moderated her diet to avoid raw sugar and simple carbohydrates, and her big tumors shrank down accordingly. But the fact that her body holds onto sugar — any sugar — for more than two hours before her cells can fully absorb the incoming supply still leaves her vulnerable to sugar as follows:

Diabetes, a condition where *glucose* (sugar) from digested food is not absorbed by the body's cells in a timely manner, results in a buildup of sugar in your bloodstream. It is important to understand the causes of diabetes and the fallout from this condition as it pertains, in my opinion, to cancer.

Once the body breaks down incoming food into the "bite-sized" glucose sugar molecules that cells can absorb, the absorption process requires an escort molecule called *insulin* to bring the glucose to the cell. The insulin molecule is created by the pancreas, which squirts various useful enzymes, including insulin, into the digestive tract for absorption into the bloodstream.

Once in the bloodstream, insulin molecules first bind with glucose molecules, essentially grabbing onto the sugar floating in the blood plasma, and next attach themselves to insulin-specific receptors on cell walls allowing the cells to take possession of the sugar just brought to them.

When you "have diabetes," either your pancreas is not making enough of these insulin transporter molecules (Type 1 diabetes), or over time, your cell receptors have become insensitive to the insulin molecule and are not binding to it at the needed rate (Type 2 diabetes).

Or, you could have both conditions in play — insufficient insulin production and enfeebled cell receptors — both the result of genetic weakness, pancreatic infection, and or age. Through whichever cause, too much sugar effectively corrodes exposed elements of the body's infrastructure — for example, blood vessels, nerves, and skin — leading to conditions like heart disease and blindness.

Whatever the Type 1 or Type 2 combination, with diabetes, trillions of cells are not getting adequate supplies of nutrients.

Large quantities of sugar are simply circulating around in the bloodstream without landing anywhere — except at the doorsteps of sugar-starved cancer tumors. Tumor cells have a field day feverously ingesting the sugars to fuel their *anaerobic fermentation of sugar* method, a method needing sixteen times more sugar than the standard *aerobic oxidation of sugar* method followed by noncancerous cells.

With a cancer situation, any sluggishness by the body in absorbing sugar results in longer sugar-spike durations thus providing time for tumor cells to "chow down" on their desperately needed levels of sugar.

Though this whole hypothesis needs to be researched, for now I assume the fact that "diabetes causes sugar duration extension," a factor in providing fuel to cancer even when your are strict with your diet.

To address this likely situation, Laura added a plant-based supplement called Glucose Reduce proscribed by Doctor Brownstein (a holistic MD) containing numerous plant extracts known both to promote insulin production inside the pancreas and insulin sensitivity on the cell walls. To measure the results of this supplement, Laura and I revisited the Russian doctor in Fairfield, Connecticut to measure Laura's sugar duration times before taking the herbal supplement as compared to Laura's "treated" sugar duration time measured thirty minutes after taking the supplement.

First, we ran a baseline metabolic test without taking the supplement to determine Laura's normal metabolism rate. You start the test on an empty stomach. Next, you drink sugar water, and over the next two hours the sugar levels in the blood are measured by pricking the finger and finding the blood's sugar level using standard diabetes measurement kits.

In Laura's normal state test, her sugar reading started at 90, rose to 130, and then to 158, and at the two-hour mark, ended at 120. Most people's result would have the last reading falling back down around 90 as the ingested sugar would by then be absorbed by the body's muscle cells and organs. In Laura's case, sugar was still circulating.

A week later, we ran the same test, but this time Laura ingested the supplement thirty minutes before drinking the sugar water. This time, her final number came down to 95 rather than 120. This showed that the supplement indeed caused the cellular membranes to be more effective in connecting to insulin and were able to draw in the circulating sugar at a more standard rate.

The Glucose Reduce supplement contains six to seven herbs known from centuries of traditional medicine to cause this result. I do not know why cellular insulin receptors come alive once in the presence of these herbal compounds, but they obviously do come alive. Anyone with cancer or diabetes should look into the supplement and into experimenting with metabolic testing.

Putting Cancer to Sleep

After pinning down the blood sugar connection to sustaining cancer, I decided to dig into the whole ONCOBLOT phenomena. Who was behind ONCOBLOT, and what else could their inventions teach me? Here is what I found.

How an Organic Compound in Green Tea
Blocks the ENOX2 Receptor

Earlier chapters described the vast chemical operation transpiring inside and outside of cells and introduced how "receptors" on cell wall membranes grab onto various organic molecules circulating around the bloodstream. The "keys," the circulating molecules—like nutrients, oxygen, hormones, and enzymes—have specific "lock" receptors that they match up with opening access to the cell. These receptor connections serve two macro purposes: First, they provide paths into the cell for the raw materials needed to nourish the cell; and second, they provide the cell with a communications channel back to the body. (NOTE: Incoming communication molecules that couple with receptors for the purpose of directing cellular behavior are called *hormones*.)

Let's first cover hormones. Understand that the cells of the body do not have minds of their own; instead, *hormones* govern cellular behavior. *Hormones* are the way the body directs the cell. Likewise, cells communicate with the body by releasing their own hormonal beacons such as distress calls when under duress from oxidative stress, hunger, damage, and disease. In addition to the receptors designed to deliver nutrients, other specialized receptors focus on the exchange of hormonal signals.

As a reminder, in the "Boosting the Immune System" chapter, a great deal was said about how the various immune agents—T-cells, antibodies, macrophages, and so on—coordinate their efforts through hormonal signaling receptors and how B-cells memorize the receptor shapes of invading viruses, bacteria, fungi, and parasites so that immune cells know how to invade the invaders. The world of receptors seems a vast language of brail-like molecular receptacles looking for their incoming counterpart.

Cell division and programmed cell death, called *mitosis* and *apoptosis*, are key communication examples of receptor connectivity where from outside the cell, special incoming hormones direct the cell on what it is to do: *divide* or *die*.

From everything I have read, no one offers a theory on which cells are told to divide and which cells are told to die. But though there are unknowns in the science of this *divide/die* determination, certain *divide/die* hormonal interactions between the body and the cells have been uncovered in recent years, and these discoveries have led to an understanding of the EONX receptor, the receptor configured to receive the *divide/die* hormones.

Many standard receptor designs reside within each cell's DNA library. Cells choose to grow only the receptors they need from the complete inventory; for example, heart cells have different receptor requirements than do bone cells. When a cell divides, to maintain its cell type, offspring cells reach into the DNA library and switch on the same receptors used by the prior generation. One of the DNA designs, the ENOX gene, holds the blueprint for recognizing incoming *divide/die* hormonal commands. In recent years, it was discovered that the ENOX gene is implemented with either ENOX1 or ENOX2 switch-setting options.

Generally, our young cells are born switched to generate ENOX1 receptors, which detect normal cell *division/death* hormonal signals. These normal cells with ENOX1 receptors are able to register *die* signals as well as *grow and divide* signals coming from the body. In our youth, as cells divide, new cells emerge with these healthy ENOX1 receptors.

Conversely, the "evil" ENOX2 receptor variation appears only on cancer cell walls. This cancer-serving ENOX2 option forms a certain type of receptor that only recognizes hormonal signals telling the cell to *grow and divide*. Because cancer cells only listen to ENOX2 inputs, which solely command *division,* and not to the *die* signals also present in the bloodstream, cancer cells are never directed to die. As a result, like viruses, properly fed cancer cells never die; instead, they need to be killed through other means: starvation, poison, radiation, or immune system attacks, and so on.

As a footnote, it makes you wonder why our bodies formulate the ENOX2 receptor in the first place as it defies the laws of natural selection. I suppose that with most cancer deaths occurring past fifty years of age with the "victim" already beyond reproductive years, the destructive ENOX2 trait has already been passed to the next generation long before cancer has taken its toll on the parent. Hence, the trait is never weeded out of the population.

So....We all have to live with this ENOX2 gene sitting within our human DNA library, somewhat like inheriting "original sin" from Adam. Get used to it: We all carry the ability to have our ENOX genes switched to this evil number 2 setting during cell division when all the switches are set.

What Should Be Done with this New Insight?

Recently, some smart researchers at Purdue, Doctors James and Dorothy Morre, figured out an *infiltration* scheme that tricks the special ENOX2 receptors into latching onto diversionary molecules, plugging the receptor, and leaving the incoming *grow* and *divide* hormones no place to land. Thus blocked at the receptor gateway, *grow* and *divide* signals never reach the cancer cell's nucleus. And, once the cancer cell is no longer ordered to *grow* and *divide* by the presence of ENOX2-delivered hormones, the cancer cell just sits there, does nothing, and begins to die of inactivity. With no agenda of its own, only able to react to hormone directives, the cancer cell is effectively put to sleep (*permanent* sleep).

OK, I like it! Let's look deeper.

The question: So what diversionary molecule out there fits the bill of matching up with and messing up the degenerate ENOX2 receptacles?

The answer: *Green tea molecules!*

Actually, the researchers found that by adding a tiny amount of chili pepper to the tea (in a 1:25 ratio), the matchup between cancer cell receptors and the derived tea/pepper compound is quite complete: ENOX2 cancer cell receptors are clogged, smothered, and ultimately denied their precious supply of incoming *grow* and *divide* hormones. "Smothering the ENOC2 receptors" is the keystone idea, but there is more to understand about this infiltration tactic against cancer before one tries it out, as follows.

Like any living thing, cancer cells are resourceful. Even if you deprive them for a while, but then give them an out even for just a short time, they hang tough and live to fight another day. In this regard, the issue with green tea compounds is twofold: 1) To do the job, you needs to drink 100 cups of tea each day to get enough of the tea's active clogging molecules into your system, and 2) because the tea molecule is temporary in effect (water soluble) one needs to drink the 100 cups of tea 24/7 to keep the cancer cells smothered at all times.

Not happening!

In laboratory tests, cancer cells need to be deprived of ENOX2-delivered hormones for 72 hours before they show signs of surrendering (dying). You should consider a long-siege approach with this tactic, say 3 to 6 months in duration. Yet no one can drink 100 cups of tea a day for months on end.

To make this plan practical, the researchers packaged a high concentration of the green tea/pepper compound into a capsule called CAPSOL-T—each capsule containing 16 cups of the green tea compound with only slight traces of caffeine. These are taken every four hours. To bridge the eight-hour sleep gap, a "slow release" sister capsule called CAPSOL-TSR disperses the compound over eight hours. Nice job!

In one clinical test, 40 individuals who tested positive for traces of cancer using the OCONOBLOT test (described in an earlier chapter) followed the tea plan with 38 of the 40 ultimately obtaining clean OCONOBLOT test results.

A second footnote goes back to my theory on the root cause of cancer: viruses sometimes modify normal cells during cell division. Yet according to ENOX2 findings, the virus may only need to influence a switch, not the whole cell—like having the new cell become an ENOX2 receptor cell rather than an ENOX1 receptor cell. The newly made cancer cell then grows ENOX2 receptors on its membrane wall, not a big deal, since this is an option within its DNA library.

That a simple genetic switch setting can make a newly divided cell impervious to "die" signals without destabilizing the cell's overall makeup makes formation of cancer in this manner a way less mysterious phenomenon than alternative explanations—like "spontaneous mutation" of the DNA itself.

Hence colon cells remain colon cells but with ENOX2 receptors; breast cells stay breast cells but now grow ENOX2 receptors; and so forth across the 100 types of cancer cells known to science.

BTW, the patented OCONOBLOT test itself (also invented by the Morres) works by dissecting the ENOX2 discharges released by cancer cell receptors into the blood serum as follows.

Although all cancers emit traces of the ENOX2 receptor into the blood serum, each cancer cell type slightly modifies the ENOX2 receptor at the molecular level leaving a signature marker behind for each cancer type. The marker is used by the testing lab to categorize the cancer as breast, lung, colon, and so on.

Finally, though green tea is ingested daily in the Orient at much lower concentrations then the green tea/pepper supplement capsules, it manifestly works to some degree in the general population as the incidences of cancer in green tea-drinking cultures is notably less than in those cultures not following the practice (the same with chili pepper eaters). And recall that besides the receptor-blocking benefits of green tea, other benefits like antioxidant support (described in a previous chapter) are included on the "Green Tea Menu."

What Do these Combined Green Tea/ENOX Findings Add up To?

So far, the cancer-defeating plan outlined in this book calls for: a) starving cancer through *diet*, that is, depriving it of sugar; b) by *immune system empowerment, that is,* boosting the body through detoxification, oxygen and energy enhancement, and with special nutrient supplements that fortify immune cells; and c) by *tumor infiltration*, that is, infusing cancer with poisons like frankincense, saffron, and baking soda that weaken the cells.

But here, with green tea, we add a new *infiltration* tactic: We put the cancer cells to sleep. I like it. A lot!

With that said, I mark the end of the journal though a few other findings from 2017 and 2018 are noted in the coming "Loose Ends" chapter. So today, in 2019, we continue with much of the plan though more fruit sugar and carbs are consumed along with wine than in the "total war" months of year one. Laura usually remembers to take a Glucose Reduce pill before a meal and pretends that granola with honey is fine. But considering her excellent health markers and constant energy level, we let her habits stay as they are. We take this tactic knowing that Dr. Bard's detailed 3D sonogram technology can scour Laura's whole chest cavity every six months and is able to spot the slightest sign of cellular aberration.

In 2018, Laura's good health continued with another good sonogram report in November 2018 coming at the close of year five. And as I seemed not to be uncovering any new key insights, Laura and I felt it time to publish this book with updated editions to come out in due course.

Following is a sample report from Doctor Bard from December of 2015, twenty months into the plan. His bland but good news comments are highlighted in bold at the end. It says that we did better than slow down the cancer division rate, better than shrink the tumors. Indeed, we had *eliminated* the tumors.

Provider: Robert Bard, MD,

Encounter Date: Dec 17, 2015

Patient: Patrina, Laura (31827)

Sex: Female

DOB: Apr 29, 1963

Age: 52 years, 7 months

Race: White

Address: 93 West Mountain Rd, West Simsbury CT 06092

Primary Dr.: Wayne Chen, MD

Referred By: Wayne Chen, MD Social

History: Nonsmoker

SONOGRAM

History: *r idc dense breasts alternative therapies*

Time out: *risks/ benefits/ positives/ benefits/ density discussed*

BREAST

Comparison: *7/ 15*

Sonography was performed with high resolution 18MHz imaging and 17 MHz 3D imaging including power and spectral Doppler studies.

RIGHT

sonograms reveal unchanged fibrocystic regions in the parenchyma and well outlined lesion 3cmni3cmnl.

LEFT

ductal dilation is identified with smooth internal walls without gross microcalculi.

DUPLEX DOPPLER U/E:

Color, spectral and power Doppler imaging with spectral analysis was performed on the breast and axillary/mammary arteries/veins as complete bilateral study with bidirectional waveform analysis and spectral peak at 2 levels.
Peak axillary artery 15cm/s. Triphasic waveforms noted.
Tumor Vessel density 0%
No flow abnormalities. Physiologic venous flows noted.

SONOGRAM SOFT TISSUE/AXILLAE-RIGHT

Scattered fibrotic areas. No adenopathy is noted.

3-D WITH IMAGE RECONSTRUCTION

3-D shows smooth walled ductal dilation.
Right well circumscribed tumor 3cmni3cmnl avascular and measuring 2x4 mm prev 3x5 mm peripheral and intralesioinal neovascularity=0% vessel density

IMPRESSION

Right avascular region decreased 3D-dilated ducts improved
Axillae-no adenopathy left/right
Benign sonographic findings

6 month follow-up recommended Findings/ recommendations discussed with patient.

Very truly yours,

Robert L. Bard, MD

Part VIII

Reflections

Epilogue

Loose Ends

Appendix of Supplements

Etc.

Epilogue

One day, when my first wife was doing well on the macrobiotic Japanese diet, I described it to a Russian cab driver in New York City, and he exploded, actually taking his hands off of the wheel, proclaiming: "What is for life? You eat. You sleep. You make love. You die!"

He went on to say that he neither supported the macrobiotic diet nor medical intervention. His view: When your time is up, it's up! And I know two people of high character who were diagnosed with cancer who elected to do nothing. They quickly died—in ninety days' time—without a lot of fanfare.

And so, I do not claim that everything you have just read is "the way forward" or the whole truth; I just know that some combination of the inscribed ideas and actions, the self-healing plan, worked for Laura, the mother of our four children.

Aspects of medical intervention also work, yet these doctors do not necessarily know the whole truth either. Keep in mind that traditional doctors backed by positive five-year statistics actually advocate treatment approaches that attack every cell in the body. I simply cannot get over this fact, and admittedly I hold it against them. I am prejudiced. In the past, with my first wife, in the cancer wards of the finest hospitals in New York for over a ten-year period, I saw the intense suffering of patients enduring surgery and body poisoning believing they were somehow noble, fighting cancer.

They were fighting treatment.

The possibility of empowering the body as a first step toward arresting cancer was never mentioned. Many a doctor told me that there was no evidence that sugar drives cancer, and many believed that vitamins did drive cancer. In the hospital, the patient was served sweet desserts and no vitamins.

I know of cases where a large tumor was found, and in preparation for eventual surgery, the patient was given eight weeks of radiation and some chemo to shrink the tumor. Once the tumor was knocked down a bit, surgery was scheduled for ten to twelve weeks out. Before the surgery date, twenty weeks went by with no interim attempt made to enlist the body through self-healing to further shrink the cancer. Had the patient been following elements of the self-healing plan during this prep round of radiation and chemo in the months leading up to surgery, the patient could have been safely experimenting with various diet, detoxification, and infiltration tactics. If the tumor shrank further than expected, then great — you buy more time for self-healing, delaying surgery and placing the patient in the driver's seat.

In some way, medical intervention, by ignoring the body's potential to prevail, embraces the disease without push back,, wrestling the disease on the disease's terms. The cancer is killed by surgery, radiation, and chemotherapy, but the body is not fortified so the cancer can reform to fight another day. The disease's powerful medical institutional allies keep cancer-killing strategies in the forefront. Promising young and impressionable minds attend medical school. Some decide to specialize in cancer. Some of these then specialize in oncology, radiation, or surgery. Some of these then specialize in tumor versus blood cancer...and on the specialization goes.

But ultimately, they choose a practice where either they cut, burn, or poison flesh believing they are experts at *curing* cancer. No, they are experts at *killing* cancer, accepting high levels of collateral damage, like breaking one thousand eggs to make an omelet. And once in the mode of killing cancer, statistics formulated across large populations of patients can be gathered — *clinical evidence* — to determine *effectiveness*. Yes, when proposing *alien drugs, severe surgery, or repeated radiation*, backed up by clinical evidence across populations, there seems no other choice.

Conversely, with *self-healing*, the evidence you look for is strictly within yourself. Have I got the body working? Are the tumors shrinking? If not, consider invasive tactics. It is a different kind of truth, a singular, personal truth of the resilience of your particular body to fight rouge cancer cells. *Self-healing* sits outside the universe of intervention risks, statistics, and probabilities. It is something specific to you, certain details that you can monitor.

Finally, compare what you have just read in this book to the autocratic proclamations of the top medical intervention institutions and come to your own conclusion

---

on which approach resides closer to the "Truth." Here they are:

Mayo Clinic — Researchers have identified factors that can increase your risk of breast cancer. But it remains unclear why some people who have no risk factors still develop cancer yet other people with risk factors never do. It's likely that a complex interaction of your genetic makeup and your environment causes breast cancer.

American Cancer Society — Many risk factors can increase your chance of developing breast cancer, but we do not yet know exactly how some of these risk factors cause cells to become cancerous. Certain changes (*mutations*) in DNA that "turn on" cell division or "turn off" tumor-suppressor genes can cause normal breast cells to become cancerous. At this time, the best advice to possibly reduce the risk of breast cancer remains to:

Get regular, intentional physical activity.

Reduce your lifetime weight gain by limiting your calories and getting regular physical activity.

Avoid or limit your alcohol intake.

National Breast Cancer Foundation — No one knows the exact causes of breast cancer. Doctors seldom know why one woman develops breast cancer and another doesn't, and most women who have breast cancer will never be able to pinpoint an exact cause. What we do know is that breast cancer is always caused by damage to a cell's DNA.

As I've said, I assume that there are flaws and missing elements to the self-healing plan, but I'd take it *as is,* any day, next to the medical- industrial complex of researchers, practitioners, hospitals, specialists, charities, insurance companies, insurance regulators, drug companies, and the FDA—all embracing a statistically driven approach to killing cancer from the outside rather than providing the body what it needs from the inside.

Doing your own thing is not sacrilegious; it is self-evident.

Loose Ends

*I*n the course of five years of research, I read other cancer theorists who operated outside of mainstream medicine. Two include Doctor Max Gerson (1881-1959) and Doctor Nickolas Gonzales (1947-2015). In common, both believed in cleaning up embedded toxins—advocating coffee enemas to draw toxins out—and both taught the use of diet to fortify the body's own defensive mechanisms. You should look into their plans even just to gauge the range of theoretical possibilities.

Doctor Gonzales, notably, analyzed illness from the vantage point of how your weakened nervous system debilitates the body's core organs and functions. I read his book, *Nutrition and the Anatomic Nervous System*, and it spoke to some of the open questions I pondered.

The Nervous System

It seems self-evident that nervous system imperfections inhibit the body's cancer-fighting abilities though the nervous system/cancer connection is rarely considered. Let's sketch out the basics of the nervous system and how it meshes with some of my loose ends including: tumor versus blood cancers, insomnia, autoimmune conditions, diabetes, and the use of enzymes to thwart cancer.

Recall, that although earlier I mentioned the body's *active awake* and *restful sleep* states, saying how we channeled Laura away from stress and toward rest, I did not go deeper into the nervous system's architecture. Understanding how this invisible 200-billion cell communication network operates will provide food for thought on my "loose end" subjects. Here goes.

To start, visualize the nervous system as: a) an *outward-facing* enterprise that *vividly* channels incoming sensory data—sight, smell, sound, feel, taste—through the *thalamus* into the *cerebral cortex* where judgmental decisions are made, and b) an *internal-facing* enterprise called the *anatomic nervous system* that *quietly* monitors the inner workings of the body—heart, lung, blood pressure, digestive track dynamics—all without our being aware of it. The outward-facing sensory enterprise is easier to grasp as we actually experience it continually. But the internal, anatomic system is quite stealthy as it operates without our awareness of it.

And just as there are two circulatory systems, blood and lymph, there are two internal anatomic nervous systems: the active awake set, referred to as the *sympathetic* system, and the restful sleep set called the *parasympathetic* system. The fact that two complete sets of nerves are feathered among our universe of cells is...amazing! When you are awake and on the go, the sympathetic system dominates firing electrical impulses throughout the body driving the offensive organs like the brain and heart, causing action-oriented hormonal releases such as cortisol. Conversely, when it's time to eat or sleep, the sympathetic unit backs down and the parasympathetic nerves take over firing electrical impulses that, among other things, cause your digestive track to engage and your immune system to come alive. These two physical nervous systems use electrical signals and hormone triggers to prod and temper the various body parts to perform their functions.

The Hypothalamus Gland

Sitting above the anatomic networks, an amazing air traffic controller operates, called the *hypothalamus.* The size of an almond, it coordinates the three-way interplay between sympathetic and parasympathetic activity and the body's hormonal glands. The hypothalamus resides at the base of the scull attached to the spinal cord. It receives sensory input from the cerebral cortex while simultaneously monitoring the sympathetic and parasympathetic signaling coming in from the internal organs of the body. Busy, busy!

I am in awe that so much is deciphered by this tiny thing, the hypothalamus. Besides monitoring heart rate and water retention, the hypothalamus interacts in concert with the brain recognizing the "danger" and "safe" circumstances you experience out in the world. These real-time, danger/safe moments are gleaned by the always alert hypothalamus as it "listens" to mood signals flowing down the spinal cord from the cerebral cortex. To determine danger versus safety, the cerebral cortex digests sensations coming in from the five senses and determines the disposition of these as dangerous (stressful) or safe (calming) thus setting the mood, which it broadcasts down the spinal cord. The hypothalamus monitors these signals and reacts to them. How?

The Pituitary Gland

Sitting beneath the hypothalamus is the pea-sized *pituitary gland* that releases many different hormones into the bloodstream based upon marching orders coming from the hypothalamus gland. For example, if a dog chases you, the senses report data to the thalamus and the cerebral cortex, which recognizes trouble. The diligent hypothalamus, picking up on the *danger/stress* vibe, triggers the sympathetic nerves to fire up, and it releases a sympathetic command to the pituitary gland, which immediately sends out an "all-hands-on-deck" hormone to downstream glands. Based upon sympathetic nerve firings and the pituitary hormones, cortisol, for instance, is made by the adrenal glands further spurring on the heart and other muscles to get pumping.

Likewise, when the sun goes down, the cerebral cortex recognizes that it is closing in on bedtime. This *calm* vibe is picked up by the hypothalamus, which bumps up the parasympathetic system and commands the pituitary gland to release parasympathetic hormones, like melatonin, throughout the body waking up the immune system. The immune system stays active so long as the parasympathetic system is firing away.

Interesting, but how does this relate to our health?

Unbalanced Sympathetic/Parasympathetic Nervous Systems

According to Doctor Gonzales, different people have variations on how well this whole mechanism works. Some people have strong sympathetic systems that over dominate their bodies; some have a balance between the two sets of nerves; and some people have overly dominant parasympathetic systems.

But even if balanced, both systems may be either strong or weak, or both may be over firing concurrently (anxiety), so we are all vulnerable to how well the hypothalamus directs our bodies on a 24/7 basis—for life. You can imagine the long-range effect on the body when the systems are unbalanced or weak. Of course, the hypothalamus could be doing fine, but the downstream glands, like the adrenals, could be failing. Diagnostics are complex.

Here is the rub. Doctor Gonzales theorized that sympathetic, dominant bodies are prone to develop *tumor cancers* because parasympathetic, dependent organs like the pancreas are stifled from neglect depriving the body of key pancreatic enzymes needed to thwart blooming cancer cells.

Parasympathetic, dominant bodies cause the opposite. They are prone to *blood cancers* like *leukemia* as the runaway parasympathetic state overheats the immune system causing proliferating and mutating stem cells in the bone marrow.

Gonzales's plan sought to bring balance, vitality, and order to both systems thus avoiding the cancer pitfall of either extreme while also tempering anxiety and depression caused by both systems firing in conflict.

In summary, *sympathetic dominant bodies* need vegetables, magnesium, and potassium to strengthen the weak parasympathetic side, and *parasympathetic dominant bodies* need plenty of meat and calcium to build up the weaker sympathetic side of the overall mechanism.

Doctor Gonzales was controversial not for the architectural basics described above, but because he believed that anticancer pancreatic enzymes could cure tumor cancer if present in the blood steam at an ample concentration. To achieve this, he advocated strengthening the parasympathetic side through a vegetarian diet, vitamin and mineral supplements, and intravenous supplementation of the pancreatic enzyme itself. In one comparison test of terminally ill patients, the Gonzales patients died before the chemotherapy patients, yet all of them died. Critics dismissed the whole "enzyme" concept though Gonzales had good results with many cancer cases.

Previously in the book, I mentioned enzyme therapy, saying we passed on it, and the above explains the back story to this decision. The fact that Doctor Gonzales died in 2015 before I had a chance to contact him left no one to enlighten me further.

None of that, though offsets the basic physiology of wanting a balanced and strong sympathetic/parasympathetic system. This knowledge is pivotal.

Tumor Versus Blood Cancers

Also discussed earlier in this book, I wondered if Laura's dietary plan worked only with tumor-based cancers. According to anatomic theory, the answer is yes: Tumor cancers require raw and cooked vegetables to build up the parasympathetic side boosting the organs and the immune cells. Blood cancers require an opposite plan needing the amino acids brought in from meat, though sugar and carbs are out for both, and a detoxed body is the starting point for both ends of the spectrum.

Other Topics to Ponder

In addition, by just contemplating the structure of the anatomic nervous system, I speculate that insomnia exists when the sympathetic side fires endlessly overwhelming attempts by the parasympathetic side to shut the body down. Hence, Laura's hot salt baths at night empirically shifted her anatomic balance toward restful sleep.

More, I wonder if autoimmune conditions are spurred on by a dominant parasympathetic side which endlessly drives the immune cells to find and destroy targets. If so, building up your sympathetic side, which will rest the immune system, might naturally interrupt autoimmune flare-ups.

Also, regarding diabetes Type 1, low insulin, this condition could be affected by an anatomic imbalance which, again, deprives the pancreas (which makes insulin) of adequate parasympathetic stimulus. Hypothalamus issues could also drive Type 2 diabetes, the sluggishness of cells to grab onto glucose-laden insulin molecules. With Type 2, the liver and muscle cells deprived of adequate parasympathetic stimulus might simply stay lethargic.

Contraceptives

Over the years, a few doctors told me of the link between hormonal contraceptives and breast cancer. The use of progesterone and estrogen in contraceptives could obviously drive any cancers with estrogen/progesterone sensitive receptors. Here is what I found: The correlation between birth control and breast cancer came from a study that tracked 1.8 million Danish women aged 15-49 years old for more than a decade. The Dana-Farber Cancer Institute in Boston summarizes the results of the study as follows:

Research found that it didn't much matter whether women used contraceptive pills or IUDs: The increased risk of breast cancer was roughly the same for each method.

Breast cancer is rare among women in the age group studied, particularly those in their 20s and 30s. The paper estimated that for every 100,000 women, contraceptive use would lead to an additional 13 breast cancer cases a year, but mainly for women in their 40s. If the 100,000 women were all under age 35, contraceptive use would yield only two additional breast cancer cases.

Note that the contraceptive did not trigger the cancer itself; instead, the hormones in the contraceptive spurred cancer occurrences to grow at a rate not able to be reversed by the immune system. Because most cancers are triggered once you are in your forties, there are no cancer cells to accelerate in your twenties and thirties making the practice relatively safe. However, once in your forties where dense breast tissue, iodine issues, and other age factors increase the chance of a viral infection leading to a cancer cell occurrence, you should switch over to a non-hormonal contraception method.

Blood Types

One more thing. At some point, I looked into the phenomenon of the different human blood types hoping to glean an insight but only found the following.

Overall, before modern times, humans lived within broad biospheres like the Fertile Crescent, jungles, frozen northlands, and so on eating only the food found in their cloistered world. A meat-and-milk eating Mongol evolved a different internal system than did a grain-producing Egyptian.

But then two things happened: First, to some extent, the races interbred so that today's integrated gene pool may contain *conflicted traits*. Second, our food today has nothing to do with a specialized biosphere; we grow and eat what we want. Our bodies cope with this imposed "modern" chaos, but when the body breaks down rather than knee-jerk medical intervention, we have the possibility to slowly align our diet to our genetic preferences, pulling the combined sets of digestive and anatomic nervous systems back in line.

These loose ends, of course, are but educated, correlated guesses. But like everything else human, you start with contemplated premises and then try things out.

Where are the young researchers?

I will leave you with that.

Appendix of Supplements

*D*efeating *Breast Cancer* is more than a "how to" book; it is the story *of how* the "how to" findings came about. To really understand these, it is best for the reader to read the book itself. Nevertheless, though not liking short cuts, I decided to bring the supplement aspect of the book together as an appendix to help people get started with the researching, ordering, and daily taking of the plan's ingredients.

As mentioned in the book, there are an awful lot of supplements to take, but there are multiple, key systems within the body each requiring both general use and specialized supplements, especially once we creep past age forty. After all, it is age that calls for supplementation to feed our tired and somewhat worn-out cells. The alternative, facing your steady decline, should offset any complaints about the number of supplements, especially as supplements were mainly unknown throughout Western medicine until recent decades. We are lucky to have them.

As you will see, the supplements are grouped according to the bodily systems they help most. Also, the topic of hormone therapy, not brought up in the book until now, is looked at here in the "Appendix." But keep in mind, supplements are just one element of the book's self-healing plan. Diet, energy boosting, detoxing, stress management, oxygen boosting, cancer infiltration measures, and so on all come first. Don't get too caught up with supplements thinking them a short cut that lets you off the hook.

Immune System Boosters

→*Overview:* Ah, the life of an immune cell! Aside from fungi and parasites, viruses and bacteria are the primary organisms invading our bodies, and our immune cells counterattack these 24/7. Secondly, immune cells also attack cancer cells, though cancer cells are part of us, not foreigners, often making them difficult to detect. Conversely, immune cells can become confused and attack the body's healthy cells by mistake. Also to note, viruses can only be killed off by immune cells, while bacterial infections can be killed off through a combination of your immune cells complemented by antibiotics. Obviously, immune cells are "stressed." How can we help?

Use beta glucan supplements to provide your various immune system cells with the vitamin specifics they crave. Different cell types require different nutrients. Glucan vitamins needed by immune system cells are found in many foods, but that does not mean enough reaches the trillions of immune system cells in operation at a given moment. The glucan molecules are water soluble, flushed out daily, so take them daily.

Use red Reishe mushroom extract supplements daily. The organic compounds from this mushroom stimulate immune cells to be "more alert" in going after viruses, bacteria, fungi, and parasites. But, if you ask more from these immune cells, make sure you feed them with the above glucans.

Use vitamin A in a low dose when feeling a cold coming on. Vitamin A, like glucans, provides immune cells with fuel especially along the respiratory and digestive tracts. But don't overdo it. Vitamin A is fat soluble, meaning it can be stored within the body and is not washed out daily like the water soluble vitamins such as vitamin C. But if you are run down, try a three-day boost.

Use astragalus root (a plant extract), which is another immune system booster that also contains a complement of antioxidants that generally protect all cells from *free radicals* (molecules with mismatched proton/electron pairings that rob parts from healthy cells).

Use Nano Curcumin Plus – A natural anti-viral treatment to counter both viruses and the inflammatory response caused by viruses. *Nano Curcumin Plus* includes high-quality Nano Curcumin and Nano Boswellia extracts (Nano means super refined for easy absorption). Doctor Blaylock recommends *Nano Curcumin Plus* as it has both compounds in their easily absorbed form.

Nervous System Boosters

→*Overview:* The nervous system is ignored because we cannot see it, yet it operates trillions of specialized cells using fancy biochemical compounds to do its thing. So don't let it down as it ages. Supplements include: B6, B12, folic acid, and magnesium/potassium metals.

Use B6, a component used in building chemical neurotransmitters throughout the central nervous system.

Use B12, another building block compound used to create the "myelin" sheath surrounding the nerves.

Use folic acid to provide fuel to the peripheral nerves, which carry signals to and from the spinal cord thus fostering both sensation and the proper operation of the hidden anatomic nervous system, which directs organs and glands throughout the body.

Use a low dose of **magnesium** and **potassium** each day to bolster your parasympathetic nervous system, the branch of the hidden anatomic nervous system that stimulates the immune cells and the digestive track. The parasympathetic side of the anatomic nervous system can be overwhelmed by its counterpart, the sympathetic nervous system, which is hyperactive during the day and sometimes too stubborn to "step down" to give immune and digestive functions breathing room. Hence, the mineral boost, which gives support for the nighttime side.

Digestive Track Boosters

Use a few drops of citricidal (grapefruit seed extract) biweekly, in a bit of water, an antiseptic that kills off foreign viruses, bacteria, fungi, and parasites residing in the intestines but (somehow) does not kill the good bacteria in your gut. Also take **apple cider vinegar**, another antiseptic that helps with blood sugar spikes and weight loss.

Use probiotics to keep your good bacteria level in the intestines at an effective level. These bacteria digest your incoming food breaking it down so that the intestines can absorb it. These symbiotic bacteria also make things like vitamin B12. So, to make sure that trillions of these precious helpers are on hand to break down your food, take a probiotic supplement. And have yogurt and pickles once in a while as they, too provide "good" digestive bacteria.

Use lemon juice daily; it calms the stomach from overproducing acid and boosts the metabolism assisting in weight loss and detoxification.

The Heart and Circulatory System Boosters

→*Overview:* Our goal is to provide fuel to the heart itself while also softening the blood vessels circulating the blood. As the heart pumps, the whole vessel network needs to easily expand to receive the new blood and then recede to push used blood back to the heart. Without this expanding and receding pulsing action, the heart does all the work. What can we do to help?

Use CoQ10 supplements. These enzymes support the mitochondria living in every cell. *Mitochondria* are separate organisms living in our cells that make energy for the cell they reside in. Heart and neuron cells have many more mitochondria per cell than, say, bone cells because of the massive 24/7 workload these high-performance cells deliver. Technically, the CoQ10 is a *coenzyme* (needing other enzymes), a *catalyst molecule* used by mitochondria to perform their energy generation function. Don't starve these little guys out of their basic needs especially for the workhorse heart and neuron cells.

Use PQQ. Studies show that the effectiveness of CoQ10 is boosted if you also take 20 grams of PQQ each day (PQQ is a "sister" coenzyme to CoQ10 found in plants).

The combination apparently: a) increases the number of mitochondria inside the cells, and b) dramatically shields cells against oxidative stress, both big offsets to aging, cancer, and dementia.

Use resveratrol supplements. These relax your vascular system so that it expands and retracts fluidly with each heartbeat. Furthermore, by opening capillaries for better blood flow, vitamins and immune system support agents can more optimally reach the deep individual cells. Resveratrol comes from the juice of red grape skins. For years, the world wondered, why do the French suffer fewer heart issues? Red wine and its resveratrol compound is the answer. Drink red wine, but buy the pill concentrate as well.

Use beet root powder. Beets are rich in natural chemicals called nitrates. Through a chain reaction, your body changes nitrates into nitric oxide, which helps with blood flow and blood pressure. Add this purple powder to an a.m. drink.

Use omega 3 daily. This "fatty acid' somehow controls excess triglyceride levels in the blood by parking triglycerides inside the fat cells they normally reside in until an energy need calls them out. Keeping them properly warehoused mitigates triglyceride overload in the bloodstream, one cause of heart disease. Omega 3 can be ingested through fish, nuts, and seeds, but a supplemental boost is probably needed by most people. Omega 3 is said to help with arthritic and depression issues as well. Also, pregnant woman need it to foster neurological development in the fetus.

Sex Systems

➜ *Overview:* Men and woman are certainly different physiologically. For one, woman have menstrual cycles and men have prostate mechanisms. Each system has its own special tricks to prevent disease.

Use iodine. Woman may need to take iodine supplements if their thyroid gland does not supply adequate levels of iodine to the breast and uterus. Women with thyroid conditions, the iodine supplier, are greatly at risk. The female immune system uses the iodine (an antiseptic) to ward off viruses when the sex organs are vulnerable due to increased cell division at the beginning of the menstrual cycle. You need a blood test to determine if your iodine level needs supplementation.

Use zinc. Likewise, men probably need to take a zinc supplement as this metal is used both to create testosterone and to ward off invading viruses that lurk among the male's vulnerable, always active sperm creation and sperm maturation mechanisms. There are vitamin formulas containing zinc specifically crafted for men.

General Use Supplements

➜ *Overview:* There are certain supplements every cell in the body craves. Therefore, you need to take them and understand them.

Take an **Emergen-C** pack a day. This gives you a shot of both vitamin C and electrolytes, both water soluble, needing daily replenishment. C is an antioxidant protecting cell walls from free radical oxidation burns and viral vulnerability. *Electrolytes* are "metals" used to transport electrons through the cells. Take this as part of your foundation a.m. drink.

Take **5,000 units of D3** daily. D is fat soluble, so not too much as it can build up inside your system to toxic levels. D "reassures" each cell to operate according to its genetic switches. A lack of D causes "groggy" cells. The effect is first felt in brain cells as depression, but all cells are likewise affected including immune cells. Keep the cells on their toes, take D.

Take a **vitamin B** family supplement daily, including B12. Besides their importance to the nervous system (described above), the liver uses B to break incoming food into "bite-sized" molecules absorbable by the cells. Lack of B results in malnourished cells all around.

Joint Health and Inflammation

→*Overview:* Our bodies are designed to operate while we (and they) are young. Many healing enzymes that fix inflammation accumulation, scar tissue buildup, and cartilage degeneration are present in younger bodies yet missing later on. Production of these enzymes falls off dramatically past thirty years of age, so enzyme decline is the first stage of real aging. To compensate for this unfortunate reality, the following enzyme blocker and enzyme boosting agents can be taken as supplements.

Use glucosamine to block various bodily enzymes naturally designed for younger bodies that intentionally erode your cartilage in order to spur new cartilage growth. These erosion enzymes become too heavy-handed as you grow older chewing away cartilage reserves at an unbalanced rate. Again, our bodies were not designed to last long in the original natural state, so this enzyme-erosion system worked fine with original life expectancies, but by living longer, the cartilage erosion function eventually outruns itself causing cartilage cell deterioration to occur without adequate cartilage replacement cell divisions. Glucosamine blocks these destructive enzymes slowing cartilage erosion, thereby limiting the painful inflammation caused by excessive erosion in the joints.

Use wobenzym-n to provide your whole body with the ability to regulate inflammation at more balanced levels. Generally, the body creates inflammation whenever it perceives trouble, and for the most part, it creates a lot of inflammation "just to be sure." Wobenzyme works with the inflammation-producing cells to calm them down. It is not a steroid that turns these cells off; it simply tempers their propensity to create large amounts of inflammation at all opportunities. This calming enzyme formulated in Germany and in use there for fifty years appears to have no side effects and is used systemically throughout the body, including in spinal and joint areas, to moderate inflammation, thus reducing the stiffness and pain tied to inflammation overload.

Use serrapeptase to break down old scar tissue and to release stores of inflammation trapped around old scar tissue. When young, the body makes ample levels of this enzyme, which breaks down the proteins that make up dead tissue (scar tissue). But again, past age thirty, the production of this key enzyme falls off, so rather than cleaning up scar tissue once healing is complete, scar tissue builds up throughout the body for the rest of your life.

Over time, enough dead material saturates many parts of your body impinging the blood and lymph circulatory pathways that would otherwise carry off hidden stores of inflammation. The combined scar tissue and the inflammation pockets cause stiffness and pain. Wear these down.

Use primrose oil droplets daily to help dissolve old scar tissue. Unlike serrapeptase (previously mentioned), which our bodies produce while young, primrose is an outside organic molecule that happens to work well as a scar-busting enzyme once ingested, plus it offers strong antioxidants. Overall, primrose is a good option to counter the "dense breast tissue" condition described in detail earlier in the book.

Use Copaiba. *Copaiba* is an oil extracted from a South American tree that holds an organic molecule called *betacaryophyllene*, a molecule that moderates chronic inflammation in the body. Normal inflammation happens when you incur physical damage or a foreign agent attacks the body. Temporarily, at the damage site, white blood cells secrete hormones *that encourage stem cell division* in the damaged area in order to speed up the healing process.

Like an autoimmune response, chronic inflammation occurs without bodily damage in play. In this mistaken condition, the white blood cells secrete "divide" hormones intended for stem cells, which inadvertently drive cancer cell proliferation 24/7. This is why stemming chronic inflammation is key to both the prevention and cure of cancer. Here is the research on inflammation:

Researchers from the University of Pittsburgh Schools of Health Sciences reported that inflammation activates

MUC1, a protein molecule that triggers tumor progression. Additionally, investigators at the Ohio State University Comprehensive Cancer Center found inflammation causes a rise in microR-155, a protein-lowering molecule that helps repair DNA. Further, scientists at Florida Atlantic University observed that inflammation elevates CHI3L1, a cancer biomarker that spurs the growth of cancer cells.

This betacaryophyllene molecule from the Copaiba tree matches up with a certain white blood cell receptor (CB2). When the molecule attaches to the receptor, the white blood cell returns to a calm state with the inflammatory, overheating behavior moderated or even switched off.

As a by-product, lower overall inflammation reduces the level of cortisol in the blooodstream thereby lowering the sugar response cortisol triggers, which, in turn, reduces the sugar spikes that sustain cancer colonies. Furthermore, Copaiba's betacaryophyllene molecule has been found able to kill estrogen/progesterone-sensitive MCF-7 breast cancer cells better than doxorubicin, a much used chemotherapy drug for breast cancer.

Steroids, like Prednisone and Cortisone

→*Overview:* You *temporarily* take steroids to control immune systems that are making a big mistake, meaning, attacking your own body (called an *autoimmune response*). Short-term flare-ups cause joint and spinal pain, false sore throats, poison ivy breakouts, and so on. Systemic cases include Crone's disease (gut), multiple sclerosis (nerve sheaths), and Hashimoto (thyroid). When going against cancer, useless autoimmune activity diverts the body

---

away from the main fight. Accordingly, for short-term cases, steroids are effective; systemic cases require specific medications not mentioned here.

Poison Ivy. With poison ivy, though plant oil is no longer present, the body still thinks it is, and inflammatory outbreaks show up everywhere, sometimes for weeks, until the system switches off.

Fake Illnesses. With, say, false sore throats, something like cigarette smoke may have irritated the respiratory cells, and immune cells misinterpret this for a viral assault. The immune cells never know when to stop attacking the fake disease, so the sore throat worsens.

The above cases call for a doctor-prescribed round of *body-wide* prednisone to shut immune cell switches off allowing them to start up fresh, not prejudiced by the earlier false signals.

Joint Pain. With joint and back pain, a trigger event — usually a pinched nerve and/or an arthritic condition — launches an immune response causing a buildup of painful inflammatory "goo." The cells creating inflammation need to be switched off *locally*, and a cortisone shot in the area does this. If the root cause reoccurs, a fresh trigger will restart the immune response, so after eliminating the pain you should work on the root cause. But be mindful, cortisone temporarily switches off all the local cells it touches including tendon and bone cells, so doctors are careful because the affected area can become permanently weakened.

Summary: Steroids shut down the immune response in order to end the inflammation being pumped out by out-of-control immune cells. Once the immune cells are "switched off" — while under the spell of the steroid—they usually stay switched off even when the steroid is washed out.

Anticancer Supplements

➔ *Overview:* The book goes into some depth on how to infiltrate cancer tumors to knock them off track. The tactic tricks them into ingesting substances that inhibit cell division effectively stifling the tumor's aggression while you simultaneously starve them of sugars and attack them with your immune cells. The top infiltration weapons include **baking soda, CBD oil,** and **frankincense**, but others like **saffron** can be used. (See earlier writing in the book to see how these work.)

CBD Oil

You should read up on CBD oil, a big deal, to gauge its overall potential not just in the cancer arena. The hemp plant from which it comes produces a hundred different organic molecules that our bodies selectively apply to mitigate various conditions. Hemp-sourced CBD oil does not contain THC, the psychoactive molecule found in its sister species marijuana.

Diet vs. Disease website summarizes CBD's potential as follows:

"Research has found that CBD oil has the potential to reduce chronic pain, anxiety, depression, and acne and may help those overcoming addiction. Its anti-inflammatory properties may also play a role in lowering the risk of diabetes and cardiovascular disease. It has even shown antitumor effects and could be effective in inhibiting the progression of cancer and its related symptoms."

(*Note:* Nowhere did I find that CDB laced with THC has any medicinal effect. THC-infused CBD may be good for patients near death who are suffering.)

Aging Measures

➔*Overview:* As I said up front, most of our problems come from aging. The cells, after multiplying over and over again, lose precision at each division and become enfeebled. Supplements simply prop up aging cells and do not reverse aging except in one area: "telomeres."

Telomeres are like the cap on a shoelace. *Telomeres* (the cap) keep the chromosome molecules (the shoelace) from unravelling. As cells divide, the telomeres shorten, and this causes a decline in precision as the chromosome molecules are less tightly bundled and therefore do not copy as well during cell division. What is more, cells no longer divide at all once their telomeres are too short causing things like fragile bones in older people. Conversely, telomeres that are too long somehow increase your chances of cancer (not sure why).

Below we look at the way your age is measured, and then discuss hormonal measures, which represent the last step in supplementation. Specialists in the "PhysioAge" field can test your aging rate. The bodily systems that can be tested are described as follows by one of my advisors, Dr. Joseph Raffael of New York.

Cardio Age. Arterial Stiffness Testing: Evaluates cardiovascular risk by measuring blood pressure at the heart to determine artery suppleness.

CutoAge. Skin Elasticity Testing: Assesses the elasticity, firmness, and resistance of the skin with the same instrument used in numerous clinical trials for skin-care products.

PulmoAge. Lung Function Testing: Measures lung function, which is linked to many fatal diseases, not just lung disease.

NeuroAge. Brain Function Testing: Assesses brain aging through a series of computerized tests focused on age-sensitive aspects of cognitive function.

TelomerAge. Telomere Length Measurement: Measures *telomere* lengths — caps at the ends of the chromosomes that shorten with every cell division — to indicate cell longevity.

ImmunoAge. Immune Function Testing: Uses an advanced blood test to measure the health of your immune system.

Using metrics from the population at large, these tests indicate where your systems generally stack up against others. For example, you may be forty years old, but your skin has the traits of a fifty-year old. Or you may be seventy years old, yet your vessel elasticity equals that of most forty year old's. You know where you stand, and you do something in response.

Hormone Supplementation

→*Overview:* Much of the supplementations already mentioned factor into supporting these various aging systems, but one more supplement category can be considered: hormones, though they were not used by Laura.

Hormones are chemical substances secreted by your own tissue that travel by way of body fluids to affect another tissue in your body. In essence, *hormones* are "chemical messengers."

For example, hormones direct the cells to divide, die, create adrenalin, shut off the hunger impulse, and so on. You go to an endocrinologist to get your hormone levels checked and to get prescriptions for supplementation. Supplements include:

DHEA. A precursor hormone created by the adrenalin glands that among other things provides the creation of testosterone and estrogen, which in turn influence sexual energy, bone, and muscle health. DHEA production declines over time but can be "topped off" a bit as you age. It is an inexpensive supplement.

Testosterone. A hormone in both male and female bodies that keeps muscle and tissue supple and provides a boost to assertiveness in dealing with conflict plus a boost to your sex drive. Although testosterone is considered a male sex hormone, women produce small amounts of testosterone in their ovaries and adrenal glands. In men, an abundance of testosterone is produced by the testicles and is responsible for the proper development of male sexual characteristics. Testosterone levels in males peak in your twenties and decline thereafter. By your eighties, levels are 1/3 (or less) of the peak level. Like DHEA, some supplementation is warranted.

Estrogen. A key female hormone that promotes the development of female features throughout the body effectively disappearing after menopause where it falls to levels of around 10 percent of your peak at twenty years old. Low estrogen levels can cause vaginal dryness and bone weakening, which is why older women have more bone loss issues than men. Supplementation, therefore, has a rejuvenation effect on women. The paradox: Most breast cancer cases are estrogen sensitive cell types, meaning the cancer is more vigorous when "egged on" by a meaningful level of estrogen floating in the bloodstream. Hence, supplementation here is tricky, to say the least.

DIM. Diindolylmethane, or DIM, is produced during the digestion of cruciferous vegetables such as broccoli, brussels sprouts, cabbage, and cauliflower. Besides eating these vegetables, you can obtain DIM through supplements. DIM, heavily researched, shows no side effects yet provides organic molecules that focus immune cells into going after viruses as well as attacking both breast and prostate cancer cells. DIM is an inexpensive hormone.

Human Growth Hormone (HGH). HGH, produced by the pituitary gland, spurs growth in children and adolescents. It also helps to regulate body composition, body fluids, muscle and bone growth, sugar and fat metabolism, and possibly heart function. It declines rapidly with age especially once you grow to adult size but declines thereafter as well. This leads to the theory that small supplements of HGH will prop up your overall system as you age so long as high dosages are not in play. This theory is questioned but seems plausible. HGH is expensive. When considering this, consult an endocrinologist in the antiaging field.

Estradiol and IGF-1. Here, we are on the outer edge. There is evidence that these hormones can rebuild the telomere caps on one's chromosomes — *telomere activation*. Consult your endocrinologist and read.

Capsol-T — Hormone Blocker. This green tea concentrate (organic molecule counts equivalent to forty cups of tea) described in detail in the book plugs the receptors on cancer cell walls awaiting hormonal signals telling them to divide. If the cell cannot receive the hormonal command, it does not divide. This hormone blocker only fits in the special ENOX2 receptors found in cancer cells. It is just one of many elements you can adopt toward slowing down cancer allowing the immune system to catch up.

Dosages

→*Overview:* Though I mentioned some dosages, these are minimums, and some people may need more. To fine-tune dosages, you need to work with a naturopath nutritionist who uses blood sample data to determine the level of each compound actually residing in the blood system. Supplemented nutrients are only partially absorbed through the digestive system, so different folks need different dosages.

For a few hundred dollars, you can get an absorption test that measures the levels of forty vitamins and minerals residing within your white blood cells. This test determines what actually makes it to the finish line at the cellular level. If, for example, your vitamin B12 count is in the bottom 10 percent of the human race, then vitamin B12 supplementation is warranted. A naturopath doctor takes a blood sample and sends it to the lab. Your levels are compared to the spectrum of all other people who have been tested.

Conclusion

*F*irst, there are hundreds of specialized supplements out there. Those mentioned in the previous sections are the ones we considered and chose for Laura's self-healing program. Second, there is lots to do, but only if you want to slow the downward spiral. Some decide to try, some don't. In the final analysis, we have all been told "it's taxes and death." Laura and I made our choice; we rail against both. Laura defied cancer and has so far prevailed.

Hey, why not you?

Joe P,
2019

Preventing & Defeating Breast Cancer On-line Program

6 Hours of Video, 6 Modules, 32 Individual Videos

• FREE VIDEOS •

Orientation – 30 Minutes

- Welcome — Our Purpose
- Self-healing — An Overview
- The Research — Methods
- How to Use the Video Series

....

• TUITION-BASED MODULES •

MODULE – I – MEETING CANCER – 45 Minutes

1. Laura's Story......................................*"A 5-Year Journey"*
2. Breast Cancer Fundamentals............................ *"The Roadmap"*
3. Cellular Fundamentals............................ *"How Cancer Evolves"*

MODULE – II – DIET – 30 Minutes

4. Sugars & Ketones ....*"Isolating Cancer"*
5. The Diet .... *"Foods That Cure"*

MODULE – III – TUMOR INFILTRATION – 45 Minutes

6. Trojan Horses ....*"Deceiving Tumors"*
7. Green Tea.............................. *"Putting Cancer to Sleep"*
8. Angiogenesis......................... *"Block Cancer's Tentacles"*
9. Estrogen ....*"Stop fueling Cell Division"*

GREEN LIGHT
Cancer Fighting Foods

Cruciferous Vegetables:

-> Arugula (rocket)	Lentil	Tumeric
-> Asparagas		Primrose
-> Bok choy	Eggplant	
-> Broccoflower	Ginger Root	
-> Broccoli	Endive	Sea Salt
-> Broccoli Rabe	Beet	**Mustard Seeds:**
-> Broccoli romanesco	Mushroom	- Brown, Green
-> Broccolini	Mustard Greens	- White, Black
-> Brussels sprouts	Garlic	Spirulina
-> Cabbage	Parsnip	Ginger
-> Cauliflower	Pumpkin	Cinnamon
-> Chinese cabbage	Celery	Ghee
-> Collard greens	Sweet Potato/Yam	Baking Soda
-> Daikon		
-> Kale		
-> Kohlrabi		
-> Radish	Onion	Green Tea
-> Rutabaga (swede)	Squash	
-> Sprouts		
-> Tatsoi	Lettuce	
-> Turnip root; greens	Cucumber	
-> Wasabi	Apple Cider Vinegar	
-> Watercress	Pumpkin Seed	
-> Horseradish		
-> Maca		
-> Garden Cress		
-> Komatsuna	**Seaweed** - Nori, Kombo	
-> Choy sum	- Wake, Hijiki	

YELLOW LIGHT
Cancer Neutral Foods

Whole Grains:	Fish - wild caught:	Carrots
-> Brown Rice	-> Salmon, Sole	
-> Wild Rice	-> Cod, Halibut	
-> Quinoa	-> Sardine	
-> Oats		
-> Millet	Turkey/Goose	
-> Barley	Chicken	
-> Flax		
-> Amaranth	**Berries:**	Pineapple
	-> Blueberries	Watermelon
Whole Grain Bread	-> Raspberries	
Whole Grain Pasta		
	Beans:	**Oils:**
Eggs	-> Black, Kidney	-> Olive
Yogurt - Plain	-> Navy, Pinto	-> Avocado
Goat/Sheep Cheese	-> Garbanzo, Black-eyed	-> Safflower
Butter		
Red Wine - Moderate		

RED LIGHT

Cancer Stimulating Foods

Sugar/Fructose	Pomegranate	White Vinegar
Jam/Jelly	Cranberry	Yeast
Pudding	Corn	Table Salt
Ice Cream		
Milk/Soy Milk	**Refined Carbohydrates:**	Antibiotics
	-> White Flour	
Aspartame	-> White Bread	
MSG	-> White Rice	
	-> Pasta	
Aged Cheese		
-> Gorganzola	Microwave Popcorn	
-> Blue Cheese		
Processed Cheese	Beer	
Soybean	Soda	
Carob	Alcohol	
	White Wine	
Lobster		
Mussel/Squid	**Partially Hydrogenated Oils:**	
	-> Margarine	
Beef	-> Vegetable Shortening	
Processed Meats:	-> Pre-made Baked Goods	
-> Sausage	-> Cookies, Crackers	
-> Hot Dogs	-> Piecrusts	
-> Bacon	-> Fried Food	
-> Ham	-> Refrigerated Dough	
-> Bologna		
-> Salami		

www.ingramcontent.com/pod-product-compliance
Lightning Source LLC
Chambersburg PA
CBHW030239030426
42336CB00009B/175